Time
for
Dying

Time
for
Dying

Barney G. Glaser
&Anselm L. Strauss

AldineTransaction
A Division of Transaction Publishers
New Brunswick (U.S.A.) and London (U.K.)

Second paperback printing 2007

This book is printed on acid-free paper that meets the American National Standard for Permanence of Paper for Printed Library Materials.

Library of Congress Catalog Number: 2006045691
ISBN: 978-0-202-30858-6
Printed in the United States of America

Library of Congress Cataloging-in-Publication Data

Glaser, Barney G.
  Time for dying / Barney G. Glaser & Anselm L. Strauss.
      p. cm.
  Reprint. Originally published: Chicago : Aldine Pub. Co., 1968.
  Includes bibliographical references and index.
  ISBN 978-0-202-30858-6 (pbk : alk. paper)
    1. Nursing—Psychological aspects. 2. Death—Psychological aspects.
  I. Strauss, Anselm L. II. Title.

RT86.G55 2007
616'.029—dc22   2006045691

Contents

To

HELEN NAHM,

colleague and good friend

Preface

This book, like our preceding book (*Awareness of Dying*), is directed to two audiences. Because we wish to contribute toward making the management of dying—by health professionals, families and patients—more rational and compassionate, we have written this book, first of all, for those who must work with and give care to the dying. Our discussion is, however, not simple narrative or description; it is a "rendition of reality," informed by a rather densely woven and fairly abstract theoretical scheme. This scheme evolved gradually during the course of our research. The second audience we anticipate for this volume, therefore, is social scientists who are less interested in dying than they are in useful substantive theory. Our central theoretical concern is with the temporal aspects of work. We believe, and shall indicate in the concluding chapter, that the theory presented here may be useful to social scientists interested in areas far removed from health, medicine, or hospitals.

In 1963, 53 per cent of all deaths in the United States occurred in hospitals, and many others in nursing homes.[1] That figure points up a little noted but significant trend characteristic of economically advanced nations. In so-called less developed countries, people typically die at home, at least when they die naturally, but the health practices and medical technology of Western Europe and the United States seem destined to bring about increasing institutionalization of dying in those regions.

The extent of the trend, but not its full significance, is suggested by the bare fact of the changing character of locales where people die. Nursing homes, for example, are becoming less cus-

1. Robert Fulton, "Death and Self," *Journal of Religion and Health*, 3: (July, 1964), p. 364.

todial and more medical, and unquestionably will continue to evolve along these lines. Along with improved medical technology and changing disease patterns, hospitals, too, are assuming a new look. Whereas they used to be either custodial institutions or places where the poor were taken to die, during the past three decades they have increasingly evolved into workshops where complete or partial recovery from illness can be achieved. In turn, medical progress has also altered the patterns of disease: chronic illness, rather than acute illness, now predominates. This and the increasingly medical character of hospitals have transformed the medical care provided in hospitals. There is far less shoulder-to-shoulder fighting by nurse and doctor against the dangerous peaks of acute disease. Patients with incurable chronic diseases either come to the hospital to die, or die there because the erosion of the disease cannot be arrested. In consequence, the relationships of hospital staff and patients have changed considerably from the days when patients either died quickly from acute disease, or, their conditions being hopeless, went home to die.

That people elect to die in such institutions—or that their families make such choices for them—means that outsiders to the family have been delegated responsibility for taking care of the dying during their last days or hours. The significance of *delegated responsibility* is powerfully suggested by two contrasting situations that we have observed. In the United States, elderly people sometimes refuse to leave home to die in hospitals, and their families often concur in the decision; but, when the progress of dying involves intricate nursing care or extreme deterioration of bodily functions, the dying person is likely to be sent off to a hospital or nursing home when the family simply can no longer endure the situation. Quite aside from simple abandonment of the dying to strangers, the family may even yield to hospitals and nursing homes all but small amounts of responsibility for action taken during the dying person's last hours, agreeing sometimes to rules that restrict visiting and even lead to their absence at the moment of death. In contrast, families in countries like Greece, Malaya, and Italy frequently still request or insist that their dying relatives be moved from hospital to home when near point of death.

The delegation of responsibility, whether partial or total, is of immense importance for everyone concerned: for patients, families, and, of course, for the hospital staffs. The last take their responsibilities with the utmost seriousness, in accordance with the directives of professional practice and the dictates of conscience. But close scrutiny of terminal care quickly suggests that only the more strictly medical or technical aspects are professionalized.

As we noted in an earlier volume,[2] the training of physicians and nurses equips them principally for the technical aspects of dealing with illness. Medical students learn not to kill patients through error, and to save lives through diagnosis and treatment. But their teachers put little or no emphasis on how to talk with dying patients; how—or whether—to disclose an impending death; or even how to approach the subject with the wives, husbands, children, and parents of the dying. Similarly, students of nursing are taught how to give nursing care to terminal patients, as well as how to give "post-mortem care." But the psychological aspects of dealing with the dying and their families are virtually absent from training. Hence, although physicians and nurses are highly skilled at handling the bodies of terminal patients, their behavior to them otherwise is actually outside the province of professional standards. Much, if not most, nontechnical conduct toward, and in the presence of, dying patients and their families is profoundly influenced by "common sense" assumptions, essentially untouched by professional or even rational considerations or by current advancement in social-psychological knowledge.

It is also important that the institutionalization of terminal care occurs within a place of work—for such care is "work" where usually the hospital staff must give care simultaneously to dying *and* recovering patients. Even casual scrutiny of terminal care from the perspective of work shows that the staff's conditions of work can profoundly affect the specific care they provide. Although

2. *Awareness of Dying* (Chicago: Aldine Publishing Company, 1965).

professional canons govern the more technical aspects of such care, even those are far from unaffected by the nature of the hospital as an organization for work.

It is safe to predict that the shift in delegation of responsibility from family to hospitals, nursing homes, and other institutions yet to be invented will bring about an increasing examination of what happens as patients lie dying in those institutions—what happens not only to patients but to everyone implicated in the dying. We conceive of this book as a venture in this exploration. It carries one step farther our previous examination of hospitalized terminal care in *Awareness of Dying*. In that book, we focused upon the consequences of who did or did not recognize that the patient was dying. In the present book, the emphasis is on dying as a *temporal process*; "awareness" is a secondary consideration.

However swiftly some deaths may come, each takes place "over time," frequently over quite a bit of time. Since the speed of dying and the events that accompany it can vary so greatly, our focus on the temporal aspects of dying must not fail to capture this rich variation in temporality. It must not neglect, either, to note that the process of dying in hospitals is much affected by professional training and codes, and by the particular conditions of work generated by hospitals as places of work. A third important consideration in interpreting dying as a temporal process is that dying is a social as well as a biological and psychological process. By the term "social" we mean especially to underline that the dying person is not simply leaving life. Unless he dies without kin or friends, and in such a way that his death is completely undiscovered his death is noticed or recorded. His dying is inextricably bound up with the life of society, however insignificant his particular life may have been or how small the impact his death makes upon its future course. This aspect of dying will be treated especially in relationship to what we shall call "status passage."

We take as the task of our book, then, an illumination of the *temporal features of dying in hospitals*—as related both to the work of hospital personnel and to dying itself as a social process.

We shall describe the organization of terminal care in hospitals; and, since dying and its "care" occur over time, we shall focus on the *temporal organization of behavior* toward dying patients.

Like *Awareness of Dying,* this book is based on intensive field work involving a combination of observation and interviewing at six hospitals located in the Bay Area of San Francisco. This field work was supplemented with rapid "check-out" or "pinpointing" field work at approximately ten hospitals in Italy, Greece, and Scotland.[3] We chose a number of medical services at each Bay Area hospital, selected to give us a maximum exposure to different aspects of dying—locales where death was sometimes speedy, sometimes slow; sometimes expected, sometimes unexpected; sometimes anticipated by the patients, sometimes unanticipated; and so on.

As we said in *Awareness of Dying,* the reader who is unacquainted with this style of field research need only imagine the sociologist moving rather freely within each medical service, having announced to the personnel his intention of "studying terminal patients and what happens around them." He trails personnel around the service, watching them at work, sometimes questioning them about details. He sits at the nursing station. He listens to conversations. Occasionally he queries the staff members, either about events he has seen or about events someone has described to him. Sometimes he interviews personnel at considerable length, announcing "an interview," perhaps even using a tape recorder. He sits in on staff meetings. He follows, day by day, the progress of various patients, observing staff interaction with them and conversation about them. He talks with patients, telling them only that he is "studying the hospital." His field work takes place during the day, evening, and night; it may last from ten minutes to many hours.

The research at hospitals in Europe consisted primarily of interviews with the personnel. These interviews provided, as our text will demonstrate, excellent data to supplement those gathered

3. See Anselm Strauss *et al., Psychiatric Ideologies and Institutions* (New York: Free Press, 1964).

at American hospitals. Some earlier observations made at hospitals in Japan, Thailand, Malaya, the Philippine Islands, and Taiwan also provided useful data.

The use of these field work methods would have permitted extensive comparative description of terminal care on different types of medical services; but even more useful than such a relatively concrete analysis should be the more abstract, theoretical scheme we shall offer in this book. This scheme, like the one presented in *Awareness of Dying,* arose from scrutiny of the data, and should illustrate the data far more than a primarily descriptive comparative analysis of the medical services. The analytic scheme is discussed in Chapter II and is used in every subsequent chapter.

The efficiency of the scheme allows us to claim—again we believe with some persuasiveness—that discernible patterns of interaction occur predictably, or at least nonfortuitiously, over the course of hospitalized dying, and that explicit knowledge of these patterns can help the staff in its care of dying patients.

We have great faith in our theory, which *is* carefully grounded on comparative data. But we also strongly feel that readers must bear a responsibility for critical review. We expect that they will variously agree with some, disagree with other specific points. Yet the theory is not to be refuted, wholly or in part, simply because it does not always fit some readers' experiences. The applicability of a general theory like ours requires that readers make the necessary corrections, adjustments, and other qualifications specific to each hospital under consideration.[4] An effective theory is capable of such qualifying elaboration, and indeed should lend itself readily

4. As we have remarked in *The Discovery of Grounded Theory* (Chicago: Aldine Publishing Company, 1967): *"The researcher and his readers . . . share a joint responsibility.* The researcher ought to provide sufficiently clear statements of theory and description so that readers can carefully assess the credibility of the theoretical framework he offers. A cardinal rule for the researcher is that whenever he himself feels most dubious about an important interpretation—or foresees that readers may well be dubious—then he should specify quite explicitly upon what kinds of data his interpretation rests. The parallel rule for readers is that they should demand explicitness about important interpretations, but if the researcher has not supplied the information then they should assess his interpretations from whatever indirect evidence may be available." (See pp. 232–33).

to the alert reader's critical qualification. If some readers are motivated by our theory to engage in research on the temporal features of dying, we should both anticipate and be delighted at their transcending incorporation of our own work.

Time for Dying is the third of a series of four monographs resulting from a six-year research program financed by the National Institute of Health, Nursing Research Branch, titled "Hospital Personnel, Nursing Care and Dying Patients, NU 00047." The first was our *Awareness of Dying* (Chicago: Aldine Publishing Company, 1965). The second monograph, by our associate Jeanne Quint, was *The Nurse and the Dying Patient* (New York: Macmillan, 1967). Another volume, *The Discovery of Grounded Theory* (Chicago: Aldine Publishing Company, 1967), explains the underpinning for our work on this subject. The final monograph will be a long case study about a single patient, in which the theory presented in the previously published monographs is applied.

We are indebted to many people. We wish especially to thank Jeanne Quint, the third member of the project team, for her invaluable and collegial support; also Mrs. Elaine MacDonald and Ruth Fleshman, who assisted in data collection during an early phase of the project. Howard S. Becker, editor of the Observations series in which this book appears, read our original manuscript and made many contributions to the final version, and we wish to thank him here. From a number of colleagues we received general support and specific commentary, especially in the writing of this book: Fred Davis, Louis Schaw, Leonard Schatzman, Helen Nahm, Mrs. Mildred McIntyre, Jeanne Hallburg, Mrs. Shizuko Fagerhaugh and Mrs. Shirley Teale. We would like also to thank those of our medical and nursing colleagues, who by their responses to the previous substantive volumes published in this series have led us to believe that our work will be useful to their respective professions. Like all field researchers, we are especially indebted to many persons who worked at the field-work locales. They are far too many to cite by name, but we wish at least to express our gratitude to them and their institutions: especially

Moffitt Hospital (University of California Medical Center, San Francisco); Providence Hospital, Oakland; the Veterans Administration Hospital at Oakland; the Napa State Mental Hospital; the San Francisco General Hospital, and Highland Hospital in Oakland. Dr. Strauss wishes also to express his appreciation to several people overseas . . . who gave us invaluable aid: Christina Papargirion and Sophia Kaphropoulos, Red Cross School of Nursing, Athens; Miss Colon Ilya and the Dean of the Red Cross School of Nursing, Rome; Dr. A. Gerola, Siena, Italy; and Mrs. Stephanson, Dean of the School of Nursing, University of Edin- *and* recovering patients. Even casual scrutiny of terminal care burgh, Edinburgh, Scotland; Dr. Cicely Saunders, London.

Mrs. Kathleen Williams helped to type first draft manuscript. Mrs. Elaine McLarin deserves more thanks than we can express on paper for shepherding the manuscript from its beginning to its end.

TIME FOR DYING

Dying Trajectories and the Organization of Work

Any study of dying—not merely of death, the end of dying—must take into consideration the fact that dying takes time. In hospitals where death is a common occurrence, the staff's work is organized in accordance with expectation that dying will take a longer or shorter time. Sometimes the organization of hospital work fits an individual patient's course of dying—his "dying trajectory"—but at other times the work pattern is, at least in some respects, out of step with the dying process. Here we will discuss the most general features of this interplay between the organization of work and the temporality of dying.

TEMPORAL FEATURES OF TERMINAL CARE

When not entirely medical or technical, most writings about terminal care focus on the psychological or ethical aspects of behavior toward dying persons.[1] Those emphases flow from the psychological, and often ethical, difficulties that accompany death and dying. However, much of the behavior of people toward the dying may be just as legitimately viewed as *work*. This is as true when a person dies at home as when he dies in the hospital. Usually during the course of his dying he is unable to fulfill all his physiological and psychological needs by himself. He may need to be fed, bathed, taken to the toilet, given drugs, brought desired objects when too feeble to get them himself, and, near the end of

1. Cf. Bibliography in Robert Fulton (ed.), *Death and Identity* (New York: John Wiley, 1965), pp. 397–415.

his life, even be "cared for" totally. Whether persons in attendance on him enjoy or suffer these tasks, they are undeniably work. Wealthier families sometimes hire private nurses to do all or some of this work. In the hospital, there is no question that terminal care, whether regarded as distasteful or as satisfying, is viewed as work.

This work has important temporal features. For instance, there are prescribed schedules governing when the patient must be fed, bathed, turned in bed, given drugs. There are times when tests must be administered. There are crucial periods when the patient must be closely observed or when crucial treatments must be given or actions taken to prevent immediate deterioration—even immediate death. Since there is a division of labor, it must be organized in terms of time. For instance, the nurse must have the patient awake in time for the laboratory technician to administer tests, and the physician's visit must not coincide with the patient's bath or with the visiting hours of relatives. When the patient's illness grows worse, the pace and tempo of the staff's work shifts accordingly: meals may be skipped and tests may be less frequent, but the administration of drugs and the reading of vital signs may be more frequent. During all this work, calculated organizational timing must consider turnover among staff members or their absence on vacations or because of illness.

With rare exceptions, medical services always include both recovering and dying patients. Even on intensive care units or on cancer services, not all patients are expected to, or do, die. On any given service, the temporal organization of work with dying patients is greatly influenced by the relative numbers of recovering and dying patients and by the types of recovering patients. For instance, on services for premature babies, babies who die usually do so within 48 hours after birth; after that, most are relatively safe. The "good preemie" does not stay very long on the service, but moves along to the normal babies' service. Hence the pace and the kind of work in the case of a premature baby vary in accordance with the number of days since birth, and when a baby begins to "turn bad" a few days after birth—-usually unexpectedly—the pace and the kind of work are greatly affected.

The temporal ordering of work on each service is also related to the predominant types of death in relation to the normal types of recovery. As an example, we may look at intensive care units: some patients there are expected to die quickly, if they are to die at all; others need close attention for several days because death is a touch-and-go matter; while others are not likely to die but do need temporary round-the-clock nursing. Most who die here are either so heavily drugged as to be temporarily comatose or are actually past consciousness. Consequently, nurses or physicians do not need to converse with these patients. When a patient nears death he may sometimes unwittingly compete with other patients for nurses' or physicians' attention, several of whom may give care to the critically ill patient. When the emergency is over, or the patient dies, then the nurses, for instance, return to less immediately critical patients, reading their vital signs, managing treatments, and carrying out other important tasks.

Each type of service tends to have a characteristic incidence of death, which also affects the staff's organization of work. Closely allied with these incidences are the tempos of dying that are characteristic of each ward. On emergency services, for example, patients tend to die quickly (they are accident cases, victims of violence, or people stricken suddenly and acutely). The staff on emergency services, therefore, is geared to perform urgent, critical functions. Many emergency services, especially in large city hospitals, are also organized for frequent deaths, especially on weekends. At such times, recovering (or non-sick) patients sometimes tend to receive scant attention, unless the service is organized flexibly to handle both types of patients.

The already complex organization of professional activity for terminal care is made even more so by several other matters involving temporality. For one, what may be conveniently termed the "experiential careers" of patients, families, and staff members are highly relevant to the action around dying patients. Some patients are familiar with their diseases, but others are encountering their symptoms for the first time. The patient's knowledge of the course of his disease, based on his previous experience with it, has an important bearing on what happens as he lies dying in the hospital. Similarly, some personnel are well acquainted with the predominant disease patterns found on their particular wards; but some, although possibly familiar with other illnesses, may be newcomers to these diseases. They may be unprepared for sudden changes of symptoms and vital signs; taken by surprise at crucial junctures, they may make bad errors in timing their actions. More experienced personnel are more likely to be able to take immediate appropriate action at any turn in the illness.

Experiential careers also include the differing experiences that people have had with hospitals. Some patients return repeatedly to the same hospital ward. When a familiar face appears, the staff may be shocked at the patient's deterioration, thinking *"Now* he is going to die," and may therefore react differently than they would to someone new to the ward. Likewise, the extent of the patient's familiarity with the ways of hospitals or of a particular hospital influence his reactions during the course of dying. In short, both the illness careers and the hospital careers of all parties in the dying situation may be of considerable importance, affecting both the interaction around the dying patient and the organization of his terminal care.

One other type of experience is highly relevant: the differing "personal careers" of the interactants in the dying situation—the more personal aspects of the interaction. We shall later discuss instances where the reactions of young nurses and physicians indicated "involvement" in the deaths of young terminal patients— much more so, generally, than in the deaths of elderly patients. Similarly, if an older woman patient reminds a young nurse of her own deceased mother, the nurse's actions toward her may be affected.

Another aspect of the effect of personal career on the dying situation is in the conception of time. Recognizing his approaching death, an elderly patient who has had a long and satisfying life may welcome it. He may also wish to review that life publicly. His wife or nurse, however, may refuse to listen, telling him that he should not give up hope of living, or even cautioning him against being "so morbid." On the other hand, other patients may throw the staff into turmoil because they will not accept their dying. Nonacceptance sometimes signifies a patient's protest against destiny for making him leave "unfinished work." These various time conceptions of different patients in the dying situation may run counter not only to each other, but also to the staff's work time concepts; as, for instance, when a patient's personal conception prevents the nurse from completing scheduled actions.

One further class of events attending the course of dying is of crucial importance for the action around the dying patient. These events are the characteristic work required by medical and hospital organization, which occurs at critical junctures of the dying process. That the person is actually dying must be recognized if he is to be treated like a dying person. At some point, everyone may recognize that there "is nothing more to do." As dying approaches its conclusion, a death watch usually takes place. When death has ended the process, there must be a formal pronouncement, and then an announcement to the family. At each point in time, the staff's interrelated actions must be properly organized.

Taken all together, then, the total organization of activity—which we call "work"—during the course of dying is profoundly affected by temporal considerations. Some are evident to almost everyone, some are not. The entire web of temporal interrelationships we shall refer to as the *temporal order*. It includes the continual readjustment and coordination of staff effort, which we term the *organization of work*.

DYING TRAJECTORIES

The dying trajectory of each patient has at least two outstanding properties. First, it takes place over time: it has *duration*. Specific trajectories can vary greatly in duration. Second, a trajectory has *shape:* it can be graphed. It plunges straight down; it moves slowly but steadily downward; it vacillates slowly, moving slightly up and down before diving downward radically; it moves slowly down at first, then hits a long plateau, then plunges abruptly to death.

Neither duration nor shape is a purely objective physiological property. They are both perceived properties; their dimensions depend on when the perceiver initially *defines* someone as dying and on his *expectations* of how that dying will proceed. Dying trajectories themselves, then, are perceived courses of dying rather than the actual courses. This distinction is readily evident in the type of trajectory that involves a short reprieve from death. This reprieve represents an unexpected deferment of death. On the other hand, in a lingering death bystanders may expect faster dying than actually occurs.

Since dying patients enter hospitals at varying distances from death, and are defined in terms of when and how they will die, various types of trajectories are commonly recognized by the hospital personnel. For instance, there is the abrupt, surprise trajectory: a patient who is expected to recover suddenly dies. A trajectory frequently found on emergency wards is the expected swift death: many patients are brought in because of fatal accidents, and nothing can be done to prevent their deaths. Expected lingering while dying is another type of trajectory; it is characteristic, for example, of cancer. Besides the short-term reprieve, there may also be the suspended-sentence trajectory: the patient is actually sent home and may live for several years thereafter. Another commonly recognized pattern is entry-reentry: the patient, slowly going downhill, returns home several times between stays at the hospital. All these generalized types of trajectories rest upon the perceivers' expectations of duration and shape.

Regardless of the particular attributes of a specific patient's trajectory, ordinarily there are certain events—we shall term them "critical junctures"—that appear along the dying trajectory and are directly handled by the temporal organization of hospital work. These occur in either full or truncated form (in the next chapter

we shall discuss the latter): (1) The patient is defined as dying.
(2) Staff and family then make preparations for his death, as he
may do himself if he knows he is dying. (3) At some point, there
seems to be "nothing more to do" to prevent death. (4) The final
descent may take weeks, or days, or merely hours, ending in (5)
the "last hours," (6) the death watch, and (7) the death itself.
Somewhere along the course of dying, there may be announcements that the patient is dying, or that he is entering or leaving a
phase. After death, death itself must be legally pronounced and
then publicly announced.

When these critical junctures occur as expected, on schedule,
then all participants—sometimes including the patient—are prepared for them. The work involved is provided for and integrated
by the temporal order of the hospital. For instance, the nurses are
ready for a death watch if they can anticipate approximately
when the patient will be very near death. When, however, critical
junctures occur unexpectedly or off schedule, staff members and
family alike are at least somewhat unprepared. This book will offer
many examples of both anticipated and unanticipated junctures.
The point we wish to emphasize here is that expectations are crucial to the way critical junctures are handled by all involved. For
that reason we turn next to a discussion of dying expectations.

EXPECTATIONS OF DEATH [2]

When a person enters a hospital, one of the most important
initial questions is "What's the diagnosis?" This question is no less
important if the patient is fated to die soon, unless death is so
imminent that diagnosis is pointless. What is done to and for most
patients depends mainly on the answers to the diagnostic questions
and its allied prognoses. Modern hospitals are organized to insure
relatively speedy answers. If initial diagnosis is uncertain, then
additional soundings are usually made; the course of the illness it-

2. The material in this section is adapted from *Awareness of Dying,*
op. cit., Chapter 2.

self during the next few days may prompt more accurate answers.

From a sociological perspective, the important thing about any diagnosis, whether correctly established or not, is that it involves questions of definition. Even with a known terminal patient, however, another important question—how fast will he die?—must still be answered. Many a hospital patient patient poses for the staff both questions simultaneously: Is this patient going to die here, and if so, when? The first of these questions refers to "uncertainty of death," the second to "time of death." Even more specifically, let us say that relative *certainty* of death means the degree to which the defining person (physician, nurse, or even the patient himself) is convinced that the patient will die. Let us say that *time* of death means the expectation of either (a) when the certain death will occur, or (b) when the uncertainty about death will be resolved. Units of time can range from minutes to months, varying with the nature of the illness and the patient's location in the hospital. For example, on emergency wards only a few minutes may pass before it is known for certain whether a patient will live. With premature babies, nurses usually think of death in terms of hours or a few days at most. For cancer patients, the time unit may be months.

In combination, *certainty* and *time* yield four types of "death expectations": (1) certain death at a known time, (2) certain death at an unknown time, (3) uncertain death but a known time when certainty will be established, and (4) uncertain death and an unknown time when the question will be resolved. As we shall show, these expectations have varying effects on the interaction of participants in the dying situations.

Anyone may read the medical signs and draw his own conclusions, the terminal patient included. But in American hospitals the attending physician is the only one who can legitimately define the patient's condition, because of his professional expertise and the professional mandate that he be medically responsible for the patient. Ordinarily, only he may tell patients that they are dying. Under extraordinary conditions, nurses tell patients or relatives directly, but this is not the usual practice.

However, nurses still must correctly assess whether the patient is dying and when he will die. To make those assessments is often no easy matter. In forming their expectations, the nurses may rely on their own reading of cues—how the patient looks and acts, what his charts report about him—as well as on cues given, perhaps unwittingly or obliquely, by the doctor. Sometimes they also receive direct information from the doctor; typically, they trust this source more than their own individual or collective reading of cues, although the reverse may be true if they are experienced nurses and the doctor seems inexperienced, incompetent, or not well acquainted with the case. Sometimes the cues are so obvious that the physician needs to say little or nothing. So, although the most legitimate source for forming and expressing death expectations is the physician, the nurses also observe cues constantly.

Doctors vary considerably in giving nurses a legitimate basis for death expectations. ("The doctor may or may not tell us a patient is critical. We decide. They expect us to use our beans.") It is unusual for a nurse to ask the doctor directly, but there may be an implicit understanding that he will tell her, or she can hint that he should tell her or give her cues. He may tell her obliquely at first, and more directly when the patient nears death. In one Catholic hospital a nurse told us: "There is no formal declaration that a patient is terminal. Sometimes a doctor will tell the nurse, but usually you just pick it up." She added: "If the doctor knows that a patient is going to die, I prefer to know it." This nurse wants legitimate expectations, but she is forced to rely mainly on cues. Sometimes nothing much needs to be said, as when a cancer patient who has returned often to the service returns again in obviously critical condition, and everyone, residents and nurses alike, agree that "this is the last time." Sometimes the cues are as explicit as words might be, as when a feeble patient who might to the inexperienced still seem to have a chance to live is taken off intravenous blood injections.

Two principal types of cues that nurses can read are the patient's physical condition and the temporal references made either by themselves or the medical staff. Physical cues, ranging from those that spell hope to those that indicate immediate death, generally establish the certainty of death expectations. Temporal cues, however, have many reference points. A major one is the typical progression of the disease, against which the patient's actual movement is measured (he is "going fast" or "lingering"). Another is the doctor's expectation about how long the patient will remain in the hospital. For instance, one patient's hospitalization was "lasting longer" than the short stay anticipated by the physician. Work schedules also provide a temporal reference: nurses adjust their expectations according to whether the patient can continue to be bathed, turned, fed, and given sedation regularly. All such references pertain to the temporal aspect of dying—to how long the patient is expected to live.

Because physical cues are generally easier to read, and help to establish some degree of certainty about dying, temporal cues are rather indeterminate without them. The patient may die "sometime" or "at any time." As both types of cues accumulate, they may support each other; for example, as a patient's condition becomes more grave, his hospitalization grows longer. But physical and temporal cues can also cancel each other: thus, an unduly long hospitalization can be balanced or even negated by increasingly hopeful physical cues. When cues cancel each other, nurses can use the more hopeful one ("he is going home sooner than expected") to balance or deny the less hopeful ("he looks bad.") As physical and temporal cues accumulate faster and become more severe, they become harder to deny, and the expectation of death is gradually more firmly established.

Nurses' definitions of the patient's illness status—that is, their expectations—affect their behavior toward him. Therefore, the particular moment when their expectations change is significant. For example, even when the physician's cues imply that the patient is doomed, as when he stops blood transfusions, the nurses may still not be absolutely sure that the implied prediction is accurate. They may not lower their levels of alertness or reduce their efforts to save the patient. They may say, as one nurse did, "If he comes out of it, we'll work on him. He only has to give us the slightest cue." Since the doctor has said nothing official, even nurses who believe the patient is dying can still give him an outside chance and stand ready to save him. They remain constantly alert to countercues. "Everybody is simply waiting," said one nurse. If the doctor had indicated that the patient would die within the day, nurses would have ceased their constant watch for countercues and reduced their efforts to save him, concentrating instead on giving comfort to the last, with no undue prolonging of life.

These changing expectations of nurses and physicians actually map out the patient's changes of status. Many patterns of "status passage," with typical rates of movement, are well known. A classical pattern is the lingering patient: he is certain to die, but when he will do so is unknown, and he does not die for some while. On one cancer ward we studied, an all-too-typical sequence of expectations for the lingering patient ran the gamut of various stages of determinancy: from original prognosis of certain death but uncertain time, through the weeks when the patient began obviously to decline, to the time when his precise time of death finally became relatively certain. Before the final decline takes place, such patients may alternate between hospital visits and periods at home. Often the nurses feel that a lingering patient is taking more time than is "proper," because there is really no hope for him. (In this sense, even an unknown time period has limits.)

A patient expected to die on schedule who suddenly begins to recover slightly or to linger—the short-term reprieve pattern—can cause problems for nurses, family, physicians, and hospital administrators. Here is an example: one patient who was expected to die within four hours had no money, but needed a special machine in order to last longer. A private hospital, at which he had been a frequent paying patient for thirty years, agreed to receive him as a charity patient. He did not die immediately but started to linger indefinitely, even to the point where there was some hope that he might live. The money problem, however, created much concern among both his family members and the hospital administrators. Paradoxically, the doctor continually had to reassure both parties that the patient (who lived for six weeks) would soon die; that is, to try to change their expectations back to "certain to die on time."

Another pattern, which may be called the vacillating pattern, is a variation on the short-term reprieve. The patient alternates from "certain to die on time" to "lingering." The alternation may occur sufficiently often to cause stress among family members and hospital personnel. Whenever the patient genuinely starts to fade, the nurses may call the family, for, as one nurse said, "If you do not call the family and the patients die, that's wrong." The family members arrive for their last look at the dying man, but he begins to linger. They finally leave saying "Please call us again when he begins to die." Family and nurses may go through this stressful cycle repeatedly; the physician and chaplain may also be affected. Thus, changes in the activities and moods of the various participants are linked with this vacillating pattern, and the nurses typically are relieved when at last they can forecast the end of the unusual lingering.

The two extremes toward which patients move are "getting well" or "certain to die at a specific time," but nurses and physicians may have other, intermediate expectations for a given patient who leaves the hospital. He may have arrived with uncertain prognosis, but is being sent home diagnosed as cancerous: certain to die, but with the "when" quite unknown. The prognoses of more puzzling cases may be uncertain on both counts.

The staff may be surprised by unexpected changes in the expected passage of patients toward death. Among the most surprising changes are the sudden death, or onset of death, of a patient for whom the previous prognoses had been doubtful as to certainty and time. Of course, the surprise is greatest when there has been no death expectation whatever, as when seemingly healthy or recovering patients die. When such patients die on the operating table, the impact is tremendous. Death is too sudden: there is no time to prepare for it. In one instance, a surgeon much admired by his nursing staff shocked them with an unexpected loss on the operating table. Rumors of negligence were rife, until autopsy showed that the man had died of unanticipated natural causes. In less traumatic instances, when, although expectations are revised as the patient moves toward death, his progress turns out to be unusual, personnel may experience a disquieting feeling of having missed certain steps.

SOME KEY VARIABLES

We have seen that death expectations are a key determinant in how everyone acts during the dying process. We have also seen that they are crucial in how degrees of preparation for the occurrence of critical junctures during dying will vary, and in how well hospital procedures may be put to work. The two extremes of the preparedness continuum are accurate expectations and inaccurate expectations. Discussion of these polar situations introduces some key variables that affect what goes on around the dying person at critical junctures. These terms will be found useful in our analyses (in later chapters) of how people react to dying trajectories.

When the staff's expectations closely approximate a dying patient's trajectory, its work with other patients, as well as with him, is made easier. For instance, critical junctures during his dying can be planned for so that manpower will not be withdrawn suddenly from other patients nor the scheduling of tasks with them disrupted. Miscalculations in forecasting or perceiving trajectories can play havoc with the organization of work—as when one or more patients unexpectedly and swiftly begins to die. Each service usually has routine procedures for managing occasional expectable emergencies, but this organizational machinery may not be sufficient to cope with crises stemming from gross miscalculations of trajectory. As we shall see, when such crises occur, the staff attempts to regain control over the disrupted organization of work as quickly as possible. Since a revised notion of the patient's condition may necessitate new procedures or additional time spent at his bedside, considerable reordering of work—even changes in the division of labor—may be involved.

A disruption of the ward's organization of work is paralleled by a shattering of its characteristic "sentimental order"—the intangible but very real patterning of mood and sentiment that characteristically exists on each ward. For instance, in an intensive care unit where cardiac patients die frequently, the sentimental order is relatively unaffected by one more speedy death; but if a hopeless patient lingers on and on, or if his wife, perhaps, refuses to accept his dying and causes "scenes," then both sentimental and work orders are profoundly affected. A much different instance helps to convey the same point: On obstetrics services, the characteristic sentimental order is one of relative cheer and optimism. When a delivering mother unexpectedly dies, as occasionally happens, the characteristic chaos that follows is a visible sign of the shattered sentimental pattern.

Another important variable that affects what goes on during the course of dying is the intersecting of experiential careers. As noted earlier, the term "experiential careers" refers to experiences people have had with illnesses or with hospitals, and to pertinent personal experiences. For convenience, we termed these illness, hospital, and personal careers. Throughout this book, we shall have much to say about the intersecting of such careers. A few examples will illustrate their importance. Chronic patients, having lived with their symptoms for a time, often are experienced in reading them; sometimes they are more skilled in this than some staff members are, especially when the latter have had little experience with the specific disease. A heart patient who had been strapped into a certain position before being x-rayed once told a nurses' aide that she had better move him quickly into another position, lest his lungs fill up with fluid. She refused, discounting his request. To her horror, he soon began to pass out, and only by dint of quick action did the staff save him. By contrast, when a staff understands that its patients may know much about the specific symptoms of their fatal illnesses—and even about the courses of their illnesses—terminal care is unmarked by such incidents. (Réne Fox's study of a chronic hospital provides many examples.[3]

3. *Experiment Perilous* (New York: Free Press of Glencoe, 1959).

Hospital careers can also intersect. For instance, on a medical service that we studied, nurses customarily negotiated with head residents to gain a fair degree of night time control over pain-relieving drugs for patients whose pain was expected to increase. Once a new resident on this service refused to negotiate as the nurses wished, for he had never been taught to relax his control of drugs. In consequence, the nurses' terminal care was much affected—for the worse, they claimed.

Finally, personal cereers may also greatly affect responses. For example, a dying patient who happens to be a nurse is very likely to be upsetting to the nurses who attend her, and even to those on the ward who are not directly involved in her care.

II

Sudden Death:
A Case of Suicide

I'm taking the best way out . . . I can't suffer the pain in the dark nights. It's easy to be brave in daylight when there are things to do and people to stimulate and distract them from physical pain. At night there's nothing to distract.

This is a portion of a suicide note published in a local newspaper. A few hours earlier, the staff of the medical service at a private hospital had discovered the self-inflicted death. The suicide had occurred just down the hall from the nursing station. The staff was shocked.

Why was the staff so taken by surprise? What events were set in motion by the discovery of the death? What happened to the ward's organization of work? And, most important for us, how can answers to these questions be given within an analytic context that will link usefully with other problems considered in this book?

CHRONOLOGY OF THE CASE

As soon as the suicide became generally known throughout the hospital, two members of our research group decided to trace the story and to follow any seemingly important events that might occur. The chronology pieced together follows in shortened version, with occasional edited quotations from our field notes.

Death is relatively uncommon on the service on which the suicide took place. A high proportion of its patients are there "for diagnosis." The nursing staff regards it as a rather quiet ward. The patient who committed suicide had previously been housed for a considerable period on another ward, where, after an operation on her back, she had gained the reputation of being relatively happy and "cooperative." Subsequently, she was also regarded as relatively happy on the medical ward. A few hours before her self-inflicted death on December 7, her private physician had told her that she would soon be sent home.

On the following day, I asked who had found her. The head nurse said, "Oh, it was the aide. Oh, it was terrible. She was so upset we had to send her to the emergency room." I asked if she could say how it happened. "Well, the night nurse made her usual rounds at 4 o'clock and everything was O.K. Then when she came back about 5 or 5:15 she looked in and heard the water running in the bathroom; so she thought 'She's up and she's getting washed early,' and went about her business. Well then, the aide heard the water running . . . went in, knocked at the bathroom door and she didn't get an answer, so she went in and found her. It was pretty awful, with her tongue hanging out."

Three days after the discovery of the suicide, the aide was asked what happened that night. She said:

It was the water running. I first heard it when I was in the medicine room, and thought maybe it was the faucet leaking in there, but it wasn't. Then later, when I went into the linen closet to get some linen, I could still hear the water running. And then, I don't know, something must have made me go in that room, and she wasn't in bed and I opened the door and there she was. . . . I let out a scream, I just wasn't expecting it. I couldn't move for a minute, like I was froze. Then I went out and told the nurse. . . . I followed the nurse when she went back into the room, but I didn't stay very long. I went back out again.

After that the aide suddenly started getting "'this pain in my chest" and feeling "quivery." She was given a pill and taken down to the emergency room to rest. "But," the aide said, "I couldn't get her face out of my mind. Oh, she looked awful."

During further questioning, the aide, a relief worker who ordinarily worked on the service where the suicide had previously been a patient, said she had not talked to other personnel about it. She also reported difficulty in sleeping because "I just keep seeing" the patient. Did she know the patient very well? "Oh, no, not really. You don't get to know anybody on nights like you do on days." The aide then speculated, "I wonder why anybody would do anything like that, and her doctor was in there about midnight that night, too." Showing signs of weeping and upset, she broke off the interview, saying, "It's such a shock, I just keep seeing her."

The night nurse who had accompanied the aide back into the room had immediately telephoned her supervisor, who quickly came up, and the intern and the private physician. The intern called the woman's husband and looked briefly at the corpse. Shortly thereafter, the aide was taken by the supervisor to the emergency room, and the nurse was left alone. "And this," she observed, "is the worst time of the morning to have this kind of thing happen. This is the time all the work has to be done." The husband arrived about 45 minutes after the suicide had been discovered. His wife's body was still in the room because the coroner, who must examine a suicide before the body can be moved, had not yet arrived. (The private physician, delayed by heavy traffic, did not arrive until 8 o'clock.) The husband wanted to go into the room. Just as the nurse had dissuaded him, the telephone rang briefly. If it had continued to ring, she would have chosen to ignore it and to concentrate instead on persuading him not to go into the room.

> What really shocked the nurse was seeing the body; it was, as she said, "pretty grotesque." This is what bothered her about letting the husband go into the room.

This night nurse did not finish her work until 10:00 A.M., when finally she left the hospital. During the emergency period after the body was discovered, no additional manpower was sent to the ward. When interviewed three nights later, the night nurse was still upset by the experience.

The head nurse arrived at 7:30 A.M. Later in the morning, the husband returned to pick up his wife's belongings. The head nurse had to carry out this transaction. According to her, it was a poignant experience. He almost "broke down" and cried when they were in the office together.

When the private physician arrived, he went into the dead woman's room with the resident. "Well, she certainly had us fooled," he commented. The head nurse described his reactions later: "He was really shocked." Various nurses and aides who worked on the day shift were told about the suicide as they arrived on the floor. (One nurse who was taking two days of leave did not know of the death until she returned to work.) All were "shocked." The nursing staff on the patient's earlier service was also shocked. According to the head nurse, they had heard about the suicide this way:

> The night supervisor was on this floor getting her morning report when the call came for her to go upstairs immediately. There had been a suicide. "But nobody here knew who. So when I first came on, one of the aides said something about she heard Mrs. Smith was dead, and did I know anything about it? Was it a suicide, and would I call upstairs and find out? I said, no, I wouldn't, this just wasn't the thing to do under the circumstances. But I told her to go upstairs and see if she could find out." The aide went upstairs and came back with the news.

The field worker asked the head nurse the next day whether she had found it hard to work on the day of the suicide. No, she had just gone about her work. "I didn't think about it too much. But when I get home, usually I lie down and take a nap before my husband comes home. Well I'll tell you, it was like I could hear every creek in the house and I just couldn't get it off my mind." Another aide, overhearing this conversation remarked, "Gosh, I would have had a heck of a time. I'm glad I was off that day."

Asked whether the other patients knew about the suicide on the day it occurred, the head nurse noted: "You know, it was funny that day. Nobody asked about her." Not even Mrs. Jones, a patient who had the reputation of getting on everybody's nerves. Actually, however, Mrs. Jones had read about the suicide in the paper and accosted an aide the next day with, "How come you didn't tell me about Mrs. Smith?" The aide, who had not been at the hospital the day before, countered with, "What do you mean?" The patient answered, "About the dying." The aide asked, "Oh, how did it happen, was she at home?" Mrs. Jones clarified, "No, it was right here at this hospital." Asked how she knew, she said, "Oh, I have my way. But, of course, I also read it in the paper."

Understandably, there was a great buzz of talk about the event among the staff during the following two or three days. As the desk clerk said: "For two days, it was all that was talked about. Things were pretty disorganized." Their talking had several facets. Latecomers were being filled in on details of the death and the events following it. Reasons were sought for the suicide. Staff members retailed whatever they could remember of what the patient had said in their presence, thus building up among themselves broad, composite pictures of the patient. Personnel were also agreeing among themselves that they could not have foreseen her intentions; they could not, then, have prevented the suicide.

Nevertheless, two days after the event, a meeting was called for the benefit of the nursing staff. A nursing supervisor who had been instrumental in setting up the conference remarked to the field worker: "I thought it would be very useful to have a conference in which you could talk about this situation in terms of preventing such happenings in the future." She had wondered whether she could handle the session herself, and so had gone to one of the staff psychiatrists, who "sort of convinced me that maybe we should talk about this particular case." Subsequently, she felt that they had focused too much on the recent case, but she still believed the conference useful, since the psychiatrist did offer certain helpful suggestions. That these had been helpful was confirmed for her by hearing two nurses talking afterward about other suicide cases in his terms.

Two sociologists attended this conference, and compared notes directly afterward. The meeting was opened with one of the nurses giving the patient's case history. Given this history, the sociologists thought that the patient had had every reason—medically speaking—to have committed suicide several years earlier. Summarizing his impressions afterward, one of the sociologists said:

> For much of the hour . . . they were reconstructing this woman's story. By the time they finished, it had become a collective story. Now they know what this woman was all about. By "all about" I don't mean they were accurate, I mean what they can now talk about. They share now each other's bits of story; and the story cannot be any longer what it was for each before. An essential part of the story, because she was a suicide, was causation: Why did she do it? Really, this is what I felt they were searching for. And the psychiatrist helped to guide the discussion that way. In fact, he set up the interaction. The interaction might otherwise have developed differently. He began by asking one or two questions which essentially asked what she was like. Then it was natural for people to begin giving testimonials, personal testimonials, about their interaction with her. At the very end, before I left, people were also asking some questions about what could have been done; but then they went on asking about suicides in general. That gave him a chance to talk about suicides as classes.
>
> His role was not only that of steering the talking about types of stories and then rounding them off with some possible interpretation—which he did with much jargon—but also what he did was answer questions with a lecture— it went on for fifteen minutes with need for only one or two questions to keep him going.
>
> So essentially what I heard was first, the building of a collective story about the woman, then a lecture about suicides in general for an interested audience. But his lecture had nothing to do with this kind of painful medical case, and nothing to do with the staff's work situation.

The other sociologist remarked that she had gotten from the conference a picture of what the patient had been like "in a way I hadn't before. I got also a sense of how much patients do get involved with nurses on a personal woman-to-woman level, in a kind of fragmentary way." In general, neither observer felt that much uneasiness about medical negligence had been generated among the staff, although the psychiatrist focused many of his remarks on "guilt." This latter point was summed up by a nurse who said, as the meeting closed, "I guess there isn't much we could do because all that we've been talking about, this could happen to other patients, too, you know."

After the session, the nursing supervisor remarked to the head nurse that the psychiatrist had placed too much emphasis on feelings of guilt in the staff. Overhearing the conversation, one sociologist explained that he had noted that when there is a suicide on psychiatric services many people feel guilt for not having anticipated it. The head nurse then said that one couldn't guard against that sort of thing with every patient; all the staff had been remembering things about other patients, what they had said, and so on—but you couldn't think about possible suicide with every patient. In fact, two weeks earlier she had been talking with Mrs. Smith.

> They had talked about committing suicide, and about tranquilizers. The nurse passed the information on to the supervisor. She didn't know what the supervisor did with it, or whether the doctor was told. But she felt she would have felt pretty terrible if she hadn't passed this information on. She also felt she got a good deal out of the doctor's [psychiatrist's] telling them that patients commit suicide no matter what you do.

The field worker's notes on this conversation conclude, "So there is clearly some kind of negligence-feeling at work, with her and other staff, but nothing of the public kind we find in psychiatric hospitals after a suicide." He felt it was also notable that although he had heard nurses wondering whether doctors could not pick up "things like that" (potential suicide)—and although Mrs. Smith's doctor had known her for some time—there was little or no open accusation against the physician, such as is sometimes heard on surgical wards, for instance, when patients die after or during operations.

There are only a few more details to add to this narrative, but they are important. Five days after the suicide, the chaplain reported to us that the aide who had discovered the corpse was still upset and still having difficulty sleeping because she kept seeing vivid images of the body. Eleven days after the suicide, he reported that he had been asked to take the aide to the inquest on the following morning. The hospital administration was in an uproar about the inquest, which had been requested by the patient's husband. After the inquest, the chaplain reported that the aide got through it rather well, saying to him afterward, "It just couldn't have been anything else but suicide."

The inquest had been at the request of the husband's attorney, the coroner reluctantly agreeing, according to the chaplain. The attorney raised all kinds of points, and the coroner kept saying, "This is not a jury trial; this is just to look at the facts of the case." Once the coroner said, "You are beating a dead horse." Two of the physicians involved in the patient's case also argued at the inquest that the woman had died accidentally (probably, the chaplain thought, because they were trying to make out a case for the husband and the family). The chaplain himself, along with the night nurse and the supervisor, who also attended the inquest, all thought it was a case of suicide. The coroner finally ruled in favor of "not a suicide."

DEATH WITHOUT DYING

In terms of our analytic interest, the striking feature of this case of "dying" is the complete absence of a perceived trajectory prior to death. Nobody around the patient had the slightest expectation that she was headed toward death. Only one nurse had even the vaguest evidence that suicide might have crossed the woman's mind, but the nurse's awareness did not lead to any expectation of dying. Consequently, the events that usually occur along the trajectory happened *after* the act of suicide. The usual sequence of critical junctures characteristic of a trajectory was jumbled; some junctures either occurred out of place or were missing completely. The actions of people ordinarily associated with those critical junctures were, then, also understandably affected. The following brief analysis will emphasize especially the disarticulation of critical junctures.

DEFINITION OF "DYING"

Even a death expected with certainty may, as we noted earlier, lack a clear indication of "time of death" and "mode of death." But the certainty or probability of death itself is based on various explicit clues, such as physical symptoms or the results of medical tests. In the case of our suicide, there never was any definition of "she's dying." She was found dead! Of course, people in hospitals are sometimes discovered dead, as from unanticipated heart failure, but discovery may not shock the staff nearly so much. This suicide, after all, involved a mode of death (hanging) most people consider rather horrible. Unexpected death in combination with an unexpected and dreadful mode (she also looked "quite terrible") was what shocked the aide and night nurse who found the body. Everybody else responded, too, although without the vivid after-imagery of the unfortunate aide. It is worth emphasizing that people responded even to the story of the suicide—some people who had never even seen the patient were very upset.

NOTHING-MORE-TO-DO CARE

Ordinarily, when a patient is brought into a ward dying, the staff defines the situation as "there's nothing that can be done to save her." The nursing care given such a patient can usefully be termed "nothing-more-to-do" care; it consists chiefly of a series of procedures designed to give physical, and often psychological, comfort. It is comfort care rather than recovery care. Similarly, when patients formerly classified otherwise are eventually defined as dying, a shift from recovery to comfort care is clearly evident.[1] As we shall see, the staff can derive much solace and satisfaction from giving conscientious comfort care. But in this case of suicide, no comfort care could be given. The satisfaction of "working with" the patient until the final moments was completely absent, as was the solace of retrospectively reviewing those redeeming efforts. (The husband also missed this chance of reviewing whatever part he might have played in his wife's last days.) On the other hand, much of the anguish that attends the nothing-more-to-do phase of a trajectory was also missing.

GRIEVING

One consequence of a death expectation that has duration is that those who hold the expectation begin to "grieve"—if they are intimate with the patient—before the actual death. This opportunity to begin grieving before an expected death lessens its emotional impact. Ordinarily the physician tells the family member who seems best able to sustain the news, expecting or asking that he will pass it along to other family members. But sudden suicide precludes pre-death grieving. The husband, for example, could grieve only after his wife's death.

Apparently no staff member was intimate with the patient, and, so far as we know, none did much grieving, at least in any depth, for her. Some were "sad," a self-applied word that suggests at least a tinge of grief.

DISARTICULATION OF DETERMINATE ORDER

Later in this book, certain phases of dying—defining, giving comfort care, grieving—will be characterized as "indeterminate," not only because they usually appear relatively early, but also because behavior connected with them is less focused than in later

1. For a detailed discussion of these kinds of care in relation to awareness, see *Awareness of Dying, op. cit.,* especially Chapters 11 and 12.

phases of the dying trajectory. By contrast, "determinate" critical junctures occur when more focused, specific actions are called forth. Among those junctures, as we shall discuss them subsequently, are the preannouncements of impending death, the relatives' "leave-taking," the staff's death watch, the death scene itself, the post-death pronouncements and announcements of death, the family's "last look" at the body, and the staff's final arrangements for the dead and his family.

The usual relatively straightforward sequence of those junctures is destroyed when someone unexpectedly commits suicide. As we saw in the case presented above, the husband had no opportunity to take any leave of his wife; he was even cheated of a "last look" immediately after her death. The staff did not preside carefully over the last days and hours before death; they engaged in no death watch, and the patient died alone. Under certain conditions, no one is especially upset if a patient dies alone; under other conditions (including suicide) everyone is greatly upset.

When the night nurse discovered her patient had died, she immediately put into operation the ordinary procedures called for by death. She notified the staff physician and the private physician, and communicated with other relevant departments, such as nursing administration and the morgue. In this case, she also had to notify the coroner's office. The resident came to pronounce death, and then called the private physician and the husband to tell them of the death. Because death was an unexpected suicide, a number of nonroutine behaviors accompanied this routine series of actions. The aide had to be taken to the emergency room. The supervisor apparently fled the ward situation. The husband arrived while the body was still in the room just as it had been discovered. The private physician arrived very late. The night nurse did not finish her work until three hours after her shift ended.

This disarticulation of what is usually a fairly determinate ordering of action continued well into the post-mortem period, when the inquest was called and the definition of "suicide" was successfully challenged.

THE PATIENT'S STORY

Ordinarily, when there is consensus about a patient's dying trajectory, staff members share more or less the same story of what is happening and what will happen—and, after the death, what did happen. As we shall show later, considerable post-death conversation may go on about a patient, especially if the staff had been much involved with him. In this case of suicide, there was a tremendous volume of conversation about her death. Some of it was directed at the question "Why did she do it?" Some was focused on her suspected or known relations with her husband, and what relevance they had to her suicide. Some concerned whether she committed suicide impulsively or had planned it—and if the latter, for how long in advance. As we saw in the quoted field notes, each of the personnel contributed something to the total picture of what this woman was like and why she might have killed herself. Most of this information had not previously been communicated, at least to responsible superiors; in other words, much that had been nonaccountable was now made accountable. The result was a consensus (not necessarily shared in all details) about the woman and her death—a collective story constructed during the post-mortem period, partly from actions that occurred during the pre-death period.

There was also a quick development of consensus about the question of negligence. When patients die expectedly, the staff does not usually question whether they could have prevented the death: the patient was clearly dying, whether the true cause was known or must await autopsy. When a patient dies unexpectedly or much sooner than expected, then staff members may accuse each other, or a staff member may blame himself, for not acting properly to prevent the death. In the case of this unexpected suicide, the staff wondered aloud whether their actions had been sufficient to prevent it. As we have seen from the narrative, they concluded rather quickly that the patient had not flashed any significant signals for her intentions, or else they would have been perceived. No person publicly blamed any other person for failure to act in time. The considerable guilt that ordinarily floods psychiatric wards when a patient dies by his own hand was, on this medical ward, either muted or almost entirely absent.

INTERSECTING CAREERS

We remarked earlier that the experiential careers of participants in the dying situation often intersect while a patient is dying. As we would anticipate, when a suicide takes place, the careers intersect most strikingly after the death. At least three such intersections are evident in this case. The night nursing supervisor previously had experienced the attempted suicide of her fiancé. (The night nurse remarked to us: "The supervisor, poor girl, is engaged to a man who recently attempted suicide. It was she who found him.") This part of her personal career seems to have lessened her ability to cope with an "impersonal" suicide. The illness career of the night nurse also entered into the dying situation: she recently had been operated on for malignant cancer. A few days after the suicide, she took off for a "rest in the mountains"—behavior that reflected, by her own admission, her own past and possible future confrontations with death. A third intersection arose in the chaplain's role on the ward after the suicide and in the request that he escort the aide to the inquest. These actions are linked closely with the chaplain's developing career in the hospital—he was still building his reputation there—and its associated reflections with nurses, physicians, and hospital administrators.

ADDITIONAL QUESTIONS

Certain other events that occurred during the post-suicide period might also be regarded as important. Mrs. Jones's questions about the dead patient's whereabouts, and the aide's handling of the conversation, bring up the problem of the impact of the suicide on other patients and on the staff's means for managing their reactions. The effect of the woman's death on personnel who had previously cared for her elsewhere in the hospital brings in the idea of the influence of physical mobility ("transfer") on staff reactions. (For instance, a patient expected to die often does so without personnel's awareness if he has been moved to another ward long before his death.) Moreover, what does it mean when in a death such as this one, wider orbits of the hospital (including top levels of hospital administration) are drawn into the situation? We shall see later that some deaths reverberate throughout the hospital—people off the ward are either actually or symbolically implicated in the deaths—so much so that some patients become "patient of the week" or even "patient of the year." The staff remembers these deaths for a very long time.

We shall close this chapter by emphasizing that this case of suicide illustrates vividly how the actual course of a death differs from a dying trajectory. The trajectory was perceived or imagined after the fact. It was only after the definition "She's dead" that, in some sense, the "dying trajectory" began to evolve. The most intense staff activity took place after her death, not, as is more usual, before. Among the important events that precipitated action were those we referred to as the trajectory's critical junctures. It is significant that those same critical junctures appear also in more ordinary kinds of dying. They appear too, although with somewhat different associated action, when patients in hospitals die unexpectedly under conditions other than suicide.

III

Initial Definitions of the Dying Trajectory

When the dying patient's hospital career begins—when he is admitted to the hospital and a specific service—the staff in solo and in concert make initial definitions of the patient's trajectory. They expect him to linger, to die quickly, or to approach death at some pace between these extremes. They establish some degree of certainty about his impending death—for example, they may judge that there is "nothing more to do" for the patient. They forecast that he will never leave the hospital again, or that he will leave and perhaps be readmitted several times before his death. They may anticipate that he will have periods of relative health as well as severe physical hardship during the course of his illness. They predict the potential modes of his dying and how he will fare during the last days and hours of his life.

They anticipate how much relative control the patient, the family, and they, the staff, will have over different stages of his dying trajectory, thus anticipating who will shape the dying patient's existence, and in what way, as the trajectory runs its course. For example, during what stages, if any, in the trajectory will the family feel it necessary to search for a cure—a "reprieve"—from any quarter of the medical community? And the staff, even at the outset, may begin considering which would be the best place for the patient's life to end—in the hospital or at home?—and, if in the hospital, how to manage the death watch, the constant care before death, and the family.

At this early stage of rehearsing these aspects and critical junctures of the dying patient's trajectory, the staff may perceive a temporally determinant trajectory—its total length with clearcut stages—or an indeterminant trajectory—its stages or length or both are unclear. Although they assign as complete a trajectory as possible to the dying patient, the clarities and vagaries of the several aspects of any trajectory generate differentials in definitions among the various staff members. The legitimate definitions, as mentioned earlier, come from the doctor. Since the definition of trajectory influences behavior, these differing definitions may create inconsistencies in the staff's care of and interaction with the patient, with consequent problems for the staff itself, family, and patient.

No matter how full and clear they may appear at the patient's admission, the initial definitions of the dying trajectory seldom remain unchanged. The staff is continually redefining the trajectory as the patient's hospital career proceeds and his condition changes. Defining the dying trajectory is, then, an open-ended process, which continually explains to the staff what they must do now, next, and in the future in caring for the dying patient. Changes in definition cause them to revise their ideas of hospital organization to help in this care, and reformulate their feelings about the patient as he proceeds toward death. Defining and redefining the dying trajectory is, in effect, a process by which the staff maps the care of the hospitalized dying patient over long and short periods of time.

The defining process allows the staff to *temporalize* every aspect of the hospital career of the dying patient. They can temporally organize their work, its associated activities and interactions, and their sentiments. Without this temporalization afforded and guided by the dying trajectory, they could neither follow nor keep up with the constant shifting and changing condition of the patient as he dies. Without this temporalization, the hospital organization, the organization of the service, and the sentimental order of the ward would be under constant threat of breaking down, and often in a state of disarray. By defining trajectories, the staff establish for themselves a *broad-range "explanation"* of what will happen to the patient, and thereby provide an *organizing perspective* on what they will do about handling the impending flow of events.

They also engage in what we shall call a *structural process*. As the dying trajectory proceeds, it generates the need for various structural aspects of hospital organization to be brought into play (the patient is, say, sent to the Intensive Care Unit or is put through dismissal procedures). Each such action moves the trajectory along, and changing conditions force other structural aspects of the hospital to be brought into play—some of them routine, as procedures for disposing of the body or for readmitting the patient, and others created to handle infrequent events, such as the announcement of a surprise death to an unsuspecting family. As the trajectory runs its course, its process is linked with the hospital organization as a structure in process. At different stages of the trajectory, different aspects of hospital procedures and facilities become relevant for the care and handling of the dying patient. These "structural relevancies" in turn become conditions and processes tied to the staff's work and mood in caring for the patient. The open-ended redefinition of the trajectory, and its linkage with the structural processes of hospital care, come to an end in any given case when the body is removed and the family sent home. However, it must be kept in mind that the hospital is usually dealing with a number of dying trajectories at once, each with various staff definitions. Hence there is a constant tendency toward disorder in the work and sentiments of staff.

GOING TO THE HOSPITAL

There is an old adage that people in general no longer believe, but that is well understood by hospital staffs: "Never go to the hospital, because hospitals are a place where people die." It is clear to most of us that large numbers of people go to hospitals to recover; it is clear to staff members that more people than ever before are going to hospitals to die. In either case, hospitalization delegates considerable responsibility to the hospital and the medical staff. Determination of what is going to happen to the patient and the style in which it will happen become an institutional-professional, rather than a personal, issue. The degree of delegation of responsibility and control over the patient is in the beginning never quite appreciated by the patient or his family, for they are typically rather ignorant of hospital structure, hospital staff, and hospital careers.

In the case of dying patients, the family is perhaps even less willing to recognize the extent of the delegation, for they tend to see the hospital as a custodial institution that is taking over the management of the patient's dying. In their eyes the hospital will protect them from the ordeal of having the patient at home and will structure and limit the ordeal of his dying for all concerned. The dying patient may be delegating more control over his style of living while dying than he wishes. When they realize this, some patients leave the hospital without their doctor's advice. But most stay (unless sent home), supporting the loss of control over their living as best they can, while trying to learn how to be acceptable dying patients. Of course, at some point in their dying trajectory, their physical condition may require the staff to manage their existence completely, no matter what they may wish.

In the case of patients who are expected to recover, the patient's and family's delegation of responsibility and control to the hospital is made "in the service of recovery." They see the hospital as a rehabilitating institution—a concentration of equipment and know-how designed to produce a cure. To reject going to the hospital is, perhaps, to risk dying. If such a patient dies, the bewildered family is likely to accuse the hospital and staff of negligence, questioning their curative ability and pretensions. This point is made clear by the following extreme example: A family in Greece sent a relative to the hospital to get well; however, he died; a complete surprise to everyone involved. The family gathered and stoned the hospital, breaking several windows. (In the United States, the family considers a malpractice or negligence suit.)

In sum, even when seen as a place for recovery, the hospital sometimes serves as the locus of dying. Its resources are better organized to handle the problems of dying, however, when the patient comes to it to die. Yet even under this condition, as we shall show, staff and organization preparations for the social-psychological problems of dying are not as adequate as those for recovery.

ENTERING THE HOSPITAL

Entering a hospital juxtaposes a hospital career and a dying trajectory. The doctor, patient or family who chooses the hospital must anticipate some kind of career in the hospital suitable to the patient's dying trajectory. Hospitals vary in their ability to mobilize the resources necessary to cope with all stages of a trajectory. For example, when a hospital does not have a particular piece of equipment, such as a kidney machine, it can mean potential death to the patient who suddenly requires one. In one such case, it was discovered that a well-known private hospital did not have such a machine (which everyone assumed it ought to have). When a dying patient suffered a renal failure, he had to be rushed to a nearby medical center. A hospital's resources—its adequacies and limitations—must be considered when linking a dying trajectory to a hospital career.

Hospital resources significantly influence the staff's initial definition of the patient's dying trajectory, and they plan accordingly for his hospital career. They have a good idea of what hospital care they can provide, and this knowledge sets limits on how they define his dying trajectory. The doctor, the patient, and the family may or may not consider this hospital career and trajectory acceptable. If not acceptable, they will seek another hospital that can, by virtue of its resources, provide a more favorable career and dying trajectory. This process of fitting resources, careers, and trajectories together accounts in large measure for the drift of patients toward the large, research-oriented, medical centers whose resources permit more optimistic dying trajectories—either longer or less certain to end in death.

Some patients who would wish it cannot be moved to a medical center because their dying is too rapid or because their physical condition or their dependence on a machine does not allow them to be moved. They are locked in a particular hospital career until the end of their trajectories. Other patients prefer a career in a hospital where excessive heroics are not possible. They prefer not to be subjected to unique machines, equipment, or drugs that may prolong their trajectories painfully. These patients and their families do not consider moving but focus on living and preparing themselves for a trajectory shaped only by the resources of their current hospital. With still other patients, the dying trajectory does not permit a move to any hospital, and they must remain at home to die. In some such cases, a hospital may send equipment into the home to ease or prevent the dying for a time, and a nurse may attend the patient. These patients experience, out of context, some aspects of a hospital career.

Moving between hospitals is also contingent on the type of dying trajectory. If a patient is dead on arrival, his hospital career starts with the end of trajectory—usually a very short one, occasioned, for example, by a heart attack or accident. Trajectories that last a few days or weeks typically do not allow time for more than one hospital career, unless a nearby hospital can provide an emergency measure deemed advisable. The patient either dies in the first hospital or is sent home to die. With their typical pattern of entry and re-entry, trajectories and occasional reprieves may last over several months or years. This long duration allows much time for "hospital hopping," especially in the search of new cures or more reprieves. Thus the lingering dying patient may have several different hospital careers before he dies. On the other hand, the lingering patient in a large urban center may keep returning to the same hospital, and even the same ward, throughout the course of his dying trajectory.

In sum, different hospitals may provide different hospital careers and different initial definitions of dying trajectories. When the patient or his family chooses the hospital, they are exercising a measure of control over the patient's trajectory—how he will fare as a human being and as a patient. The more their decision is based on experience with hospitals, the more control they exercise over the differentials associated with dying in them. To be sure, frequently the patient simply goes to the hospital with which his doctor is affiliated, and no control is exercised. Sometimes control may be sought by changing to a doctor with access to the hospital preferred by the patient or family. Some doctors can take a patient to several hospitals and so allow their patients a choice; by briefly reviewing the conditions at the various hospitals, they give a patient a basis of control over his impending hospital career. In the case of short trajectories, the only choice may be the nearest hospital, chosen with the hope that its facilities can handle the emergency.

ADMITTANCE TO A WARD

There is an acceptable dying trajectory for each ward in a hospital. Upon entering, the dying patient is assigned to the appropriate ward on the basis of initial definitions of his trajectory; and the ward staff accept him or not on the basis of *their* initial definitions of his trajectory. When the initial definitions of ward staff and admitting personnel or private doctor differ significantly, the patient may be refused admittance to the ward. In this section we shall examine admission processes to several different kinds of wards—emergency, intensive care, cancer, medical, and premature baby—particularly the relationship of the ward staff's initial definitions of the dying trajectory to the admission requirements and procedures.

Generally, we are concerned here exclusively with admission to United States hospitals that separate illnesses by ward or departments within wards. In most large American hospitals, patients are placed on the basis of some notion of an "ideal" trajectory for each ward. This approach helps the hospital and ward staff codify their initial and subsequent definitions of the patient's dying trajectory. In contrast, European and Asian hospitals in the main have large, open wards that admit *all* patients, no matter what their trajectories may be. It is harder for the staff in these hospitals to maintain clear definitions of the diverse multiple dying trajectories; open wards create many problems in handling the dying situation. American hospitals, however, introduce an initial orderliness by screening patients on the basis of initial definitions of trajectory.

There are, to be sure, exceptions. Some county hospitals in rural areas in the United States have large open wards. On the other hand, the university hospital in one Italian city has separate wards for each department specializing in particular classes of illness. Each doctor-professor in this hospital has his own ward. Some are so jealous of their realms that they pass no records on to another ward when a patient is. moved. Thus, upon being admitted to the new ward the patient's trajectory must be defined anew, repeating the whole process of examinations and history-taking. The trajectory of a patient who must pass from ward to ward is repeatedly being "initially" defined, in contrast to the re-definition process in American hospitals, where some records are usually passed along with the patient who must travel between wards.

Not all wards have the space or personnel to accept appropriate dying patients; this can have drastic consequences for the un-accepted patient. He may be sent to a ward not accustomed to his particular trajectory, which cannot offer the suitable hospital career. For example, if a patient needing constant care is placed in a ward where he can receive only periodic care, he may die between routine checks, unattended. We found precisely this situation in a county hospital whose emergency ward has a rule prohibiting accepting patients once all beds are full, regardless of consequences. Some patients are sent home to await a bed and, while waiting, become sicker or even die. Other patients, nearer death, are sent to appropriate wards. For example, a patient in danger of dying from a drug was sent for the night to the "psych" ward, where being "drugged" qualified him for admittance as suicidal. Patients on the "psych" ward, once asleep, are not checked until morning. The staff member reporting this observed: "If he did have a bad reaction there, he was as good as dead. Do you realize that just that sort of thing happened a hundred and some-odd times last year?" On the wrong ward, even a recoverable patient can become a dying patient. Another patterned hospital condition that might put the patient on the wrong ward appears when the inexperienced aide, under doctor's orders, takes a patient who needs oxygen periodically down to x-ray, where there is no oxygen supply. Conditions such as these, which mate a dying trajectory with an inappropriate hospital career, can increase both the likelihood and the speed of dying.

Emergency Ward. The emergency ward is both an open-admittance ward and a way station. Anyone may claim admission to the ward and receive a diagnosis. As a way station for distributing emergency patients throughout the hospital, this ward's functions include establishing the initial definitions of trajectory. When urgent medical or surgical "patching up" has been done—e.g., a tracheotomy on a person who cannot breathe—the patient is moved on to the ward most appropriate for his kind of trajectory. Typically the patient does not stay on the emergency ward for more than a few hours or, at most, a day. He is sent home, to jail, to a mental hospital, to another ward, to another hospital or to the morgue.

The initial definition of the dying trajectory comes after the patient's entering the emergency ward, and he is reassigned to another ward or to the morgue on the basis of the initial definition. Even a dead-on-arrival patient is supposed to be brought in by ambulance drivers or firemen as if he were alive. If complying with this rule, they will be giving the dead man oxygen. Only the doctor can pronounce him dead, thereby legitimately allowing others to stop caring for him.

The initial definition of the emergency patient's trajectory must often be established without a medical history. To be sure, physical examination—of, say, an accident patient—is often sufficient. The appropriateness of sending these patients to the intensive care unit (ICU) or to surgery is readily apparent. In other cases, initial definitions are hard to make without a history. Patients come in comatose—e.g., poisoned or in a diabetic coma—

with no history or records, and it is not readily apparent what is wrong with them. The staff must seek information any way it can. Policemen, firemen, ambulance drivers, or newspaper reporters who may be present may be asked who he is, where he lives, or who his friends are. If possible, family or friends are contacted and questioned about the patient's history—what kind of poison he might have ingested or what chronic disease he might have. In some cases, however, the only clear information upon which the staff can initially act is the fact that the patient is dying; their own immediate observations and discretion then determine which ward will best serve to keep him alive while tests are run. In the case of attempted suicides, it may be up to the staff to decide, first, whether he is a dying patient, and then, on the basis of this initial definition, if they will attempt to save him or, in effect, let him die as he wished.

The emergency ward may, under some circumstances, delay admission. As has been noted, the ward must accept dead-on-arrival patients to pronounce them dead; and it is then faced with handling the death. But in the case of some suicides and victims of violence, it can avoid admitting the patient if he is on the verge of dying. As one surgical resident said in initially defining a suicide's trajectory, "Well, if he isn't going to hurry up and die, I guess I will just have to admit him." If the patient died, he could be sent directly to the coroner's office; but he did not die quickly, so the resident admitted him. When the patient died, the ward had to process the body. The resident commented, "Well, I goofed that time." The timing and certainty of his initial definition of trajectory had been slightly off.

There is, then, a continuous flow of patients through the emergency ward. For the dying patient, this ward provides a few hours or a day of his hospital career before he is sent to a ward where he will spend more time. His care on the emergency ward is characterized by speed, in contrast to recovering patients who may have to wait long periods. If he is on the ward when emergencies are at a peak—e.g., payday-night accidents—he may receive this care on a split-second priority basis as numerous cases

flow into the ward. How he fares on this priority scale may affect
the duration and certainty of his dying trajectory. Being forgotten
for a few minutes because of the arrival of a new patient in "more
serious condition" can even bring a patient close to death. (The
army used to treat battlefield casualties on a reverse-priority basis
—the less serious first—in order to return as many men as possible to the battle.) Before being whisked off to other parts of
the hospital, the patient may get only a fleeting glimpse of his
family (unless left in their charge), who are taking what they
may feel is a "last look."

Because of its continuous flow, this ward has a high proportion of dying patients but comparatively few deaths. "Patients"
usually die either before they arrive on emergency or after they
have been sent to another ward. Indeed, part of the appeal of
working on this ward is that personnel have all the challenge of
saving a dying patient but seldom confront death. Only rarely does
an emergency staff member follow up the trajectory and hospital
career of a patient who has been on his ward for only a few hours.

It is important, from the point of view of the work and sentimental orders of the ward, to get rid of the dying patient as soon
as possible after he is patched up and can be moved. The work
order of the emergency ward is highly flexible, for coping with
all comers. If a patient *must* stay on the ward for a day or so,
giving him the necessary routine treatments, some of which emergency wards do not usually provide (*e.g.,* baths), reduces the
ward's ability to switch from patient to patient and to keep re-
focusing on new emergencies. In addition, the patient may suffer
from the ward's flexibility. Even if the staff organizes some periodic care for a patient who must stay on the ward, he may be
all too easily neglected under the pressures of other, more "real
emergency" work, with the staff switching attention according to
shifting priorities for care. On one ward we observed, a woman
with a tracheotomy, who could not be moved for a few days, was
forgotten under a siege of emergencies, and almost died.

The sentimental order of the emergency ward—one of "cool,"
speedy care—is best served by minimizing the nurses' involvement

with dying patients. This, too, depends on getting rid of the patient without delay. It is believed best to get his family off the ward also, for at this initial stage of dying they are especially prone to making scenes that are disruptive to staff and disturbing to other patients and family visitors.

Intensive Care Unit. The ICU is not, like emergency, an open ward. It screens patients prior to admission. This screening depends greatly (sometimes exclusively) on the earlier initial definition of trajectory, whether by another ward, by the hospital admittance staff, or by a doctor. Although other staff members may wish it, not all kinds of dying patients are allowed on the ICU.

The acceptable trajectory for this ward is a dying patient who, with heroic technical efforts, has a chance to recover, preferably within ten days. If the tide has turned decisively to a drawn-out recovering or dying, he is moved to another ward. In short, this ward is highly geared to the challenge of saving a patient. Next to each bed is much equipment ready for immediate critical use. Doctors are always at hand or quickly reachable for life-saving heroics. Nurses like the ICU because of the constant challenge. There is little drab routine in caring for the complex, interesting cases they are trying to rescue from death. The patients require heroic, close bedside care. The nurse on this ward is in her full glory as an immediate collaborator with doctors whose abilities are taxed to the utmost.

On this ward, the staff's goal-reward balance—the satisfaction of saving dying patients—maintains their high motivation. This, too, bears upon screening for admission; continuity in this balance must be maintained in order to keep the staff working at peak performance. Admitting a dying patient with an inappropriate trajectory (giving no chance to rescue or requiring simple, slow-paced treatment) jeopardizes this continuity. In general, then, most ICU's are allowed to screen its prospective entrants; as one nurse put it, "We are not custodial."

Yet because of the special advantages of this ward in equipment, space, personnel, and patient-staff ratio, which allow virtually constant care of patients, other wards that find it difficult or impossible to provide such care because of, say, no space or high patient loads, may try to get a patient with an unsuitable trajectory on the ICU. They phone the ICU to advise having a patient who needs "your special kind of care." In many instances this call is an effort to barge through the ICU's screening. If successful, such an attempt breaks down the goal-reward continuity of the ICU staff. A recovering patient put there only because of available bed space is dull and unrewarding. A long-term or lingering dying patient who must stay on the ward for weeks of routine, simple treatments is no challenge to the ICU nurse. And by the time he dies, the nurse is likely to be sentimentally involved and feel "horrible" about his death. This is clearly detrimental to the sentimental order of the ICU, where the degree of involvement with specific dyings and deaths is kept low by the brief careers of the patients there, as well as by the intensely preoccupying challenge of the work.

Another threat to the goal-reward continuity of the ICU is its potential use as a "dumping ground" for nonrecoverable patients who are going to die soon. Such patients offer the staff no challenge of recovery. Their presence imposes an obligation (more sentimental than professional) to minister as much to comfort as to care. Moreover, if the ICU becomes a dumping ground, its death rate leaps, and the staff must witness more than their appropriate share of the failure of medical knowledge. The sentimental order based on a balance between challenge and recovery is severely jeopardized. The presence of "hopelessness" is incompatible with the strong motivation-to-save essential in the ICU. Some ICU's do not succeed in their efforts to screen patients; they become "Death Valley," and are so labeled by the patients.

Difficulties in screening for ICU admittance is partially a result of the newness of this type of ward. Many hospital personnel and administrators have not yet codified exactly what its responsibilities are. For example, on one emergency ward we observed that the staff did not quite understand the emerging requirements of their hospital's ICU, and tried to dump on the ICU many patients still needing split-second emergency care. When doctors on

emergency learned the requirements of the ICU, they became
noted for sending the "right" patients. The sentimental orders of
both wards achieved a high level of mutual compatibility after
this period of stress. By and large, ICU structural relationships
with other parts of the hospital are in the process of being formulated as personnel work out a definition of the ward while attempting to screen patients sent to it.

Staff members on other wards are often not so amenable to
adapting. They use various strategies to get a patient with a nonrecoverable dying trajectory on the ICU. The effectiveness of
ICU's in resisting these ploys is often a function of the status of
the screening personnel. In some ICU's a ward clerk respected for
her ability to discriminate between dying patients does the screening. On other wards a nurse decides. These staff members are not
on the same organizational level as a doctor who is trying to abuse
the ICU, and they may not always be able to stand up to him.
One ICU we studied had a committee of three doctors to screen
patients. Such an arrangement is highly effective in saying "no"
to the doctor who points to the ward's empty beds in trying to
apply pressure for admission of his patient. The doctor's argument that the empty beds should be used can be effectively
countered by the committee's *professional* judgment that it is
more important to keep beds available for the "right patients."

Rotating nurses between the ICU and other wards, as opposed
to keeping one group of nurses on ICU duty, can also weaken the
screening of patients. The scheming doctor can play upon the
temporary nurse's sympathy for his plight, for, lacking permanent
assignment to the ICU, she is likely to retain more of the outlook
of a non-ICU nurse.

"Labeling" the patient as recoverable is still another strategy
for obtaining ICU entry for an inappropriate patient. Seeing his
condition upon entry, the ICU staff may immediately have doubts
as to the patient's chances, but since their initial definitions are not
based on careful examination and treatment experience, they may
tend to hold their doubts in abeyance. They are left to discover
the false legitimation of the patient some days later. The unneces-

sary frustration of their challenge puts a strain on the sentimental order and impairs the efficacy of the ward.

Moreover, once admitted, even nonrecoverable patients can obtain permission to stay on the ICU by using the strategy of endearing themselves to the staff. Staying on the ICU can be desirable for patients who need constant care (painkillers, quick oxygen, periodic suctioning) that is sometimes not so readily available on other wards. One patient in this situation endeared himself to the staff by being cheerful and by patiently asking for care only when he saw that the nurses had time and were not working on higher priority patients. He was careful not to disrupt the work or sentimental order of the ward and showed that he understood and respected the nurses' job. They let him stay.

Once the dying patient has recovered sufficiently (the challenge over, the equipment unnecessary), he is sent to another ward (cancer, medical, pediatrics, neurosurgery) to continue along a recovering or dying trajectory with routine care.

Premature Baby Ward. Admittance of a "preemie" to the premature baby ward is presumably immediate and automatic. In practice, however, staff may delay admittance until the baby has lived for at least an hour and a half after birth. An acceptable dying trajectory on this ward has this duration as an admittance requirement. If the preemie demonstrates that possibly he can live, he is permitted to enter the ward, and the staff will work to change the tide of his uncertain dying trajectory. If they can keep the baby alive for 48 to 72 hours, in most cases they no longer consider him as having a dying trajectory. He is fully expected to live; exceptions arise from complications that prolong the preemie's dying trajectory.

Delaying admittance (which we have seen happen on the emergency ward) occurs along the following lines on the preemie ward: First the preemie is left in the delivery room for about an hour. If he dies there, he is considered an "immature" baby, and this ward must process his death. After an hour the baby is brought to the preemie ward. For about half an hour he is watched closely, to see whether he will die or will have an uncertain dying trajectory. If he makes it past this period of suspended judgment, he is offered a hospital career on the preemie ward. During this career all measures are focused on keeping him from "turning bad." His uncertain trajectory anticipates either a quick death or high probability of living.

This delaying process protects both the work and, more important, the sentimental order of the premature baby ward. It cuts down on the paperwork for admittance and for recording deaths, and it keeps up the challenge of work with the preemie— to prevent death until the baby can be expected to live—by minimizing visible failures and the death rate. This latter effect on work also helps preserve the sentimental order of the ward; the strong motivation among the nurses to meet the challenge of their work is not undermined by a large proportion of failures. Their strong involvement with a baby whose uncertain trajectory leaves a good possibility for living is not jeopardized by too many involvements with those who will surely die.

That the nursing staff's involvement with premature babies is quite strong is indicated by their adoption and naming processes. Each nurse "adopts" her patients, and gives each baby a name. From then on the preemie is "her baby." She talks to her baby, cuddles it, and compares its progress with that of other nurses' babies. Each nurse usually has several babies, and too many deaths among them can break down the whole sentimental order of the ward. Indeed, as a matter of self-protection, nurses tend to delay adopting a preemie who is probably going to turn bad, leaving most of the mothering care to an aide. Some aides become heavily involved in adopting the unadoptable. The adoption and naming processes are linked to the degree of certainty that the baby's dying trajectory will end in a death or a recovery.

The screening implicit in the post-delivery delay in admittance precludes most high-risk involvements. Nonadmittance also precludes appearance on the ward of mothers who might break down at signing an admittance slip at the death of the baby, disrupting the ward's sentimental order. Mothers can also upset this order in other ways. Some constantly telephone the ward or appear unannounced, intruding their deep distress into the preemie ward. While the pre-admission delay may cause grave concern for the mother, her distress is not the problem of the preemie ward. On the other hand, the ward's sentimental order is also disrupted by the mother who does not want the preemie, for this type of mother distresses some nurses.

If the baby must be admitted, yet is almost certain to die, then the admittance slip must be signed by the mother, no matter what the time of day. She may have to be awakened in the middle of the night, the baby's trajectory not allowing her the time to sleep until morning. This, unfortunately, brings the mother's awareness of impending death of her child strongly and emphatically into focus. The nursing staff may have to cope almost immediately with the upset caused by a distressed mother that threatens the ward's sentimental order.

Medical Ward. The emergency ward, the intensive care unit, and the premature baby ward provide relatively short hospital careers to patients who either die quickly or are sent to another ward. (See Chapters VI and VII.) Fairly determinant initial definitions of the dying trajectory are necessary to establish whether the patient is suitable for the short careers these wards offer. Hence patients are quickly examined, screened and possibly delayed in order to establish their dying trajectories for or during admittance.

As the basic character of medical wards is different, so are the dying trajectories appropriate for admittance to them. Some hospitals have highly specialized medical units (*e.g.,* an intensive heart unit). Most hospitals have either a general medical ward handling the various medical subdivisions, or the basic breakdown of wards as cancer, thoracic, geriatric, pediatric, contagious, orthopedic, obstetric, neurological, heart, etc. In either case, placement on a medical ward may be made according to the initial definition of a dying trajectory, or this definition may be made after admission. These wards provide careers for many kinds of trajectories. These careers allow ample time for the staff to formulate an initial dying trajectory, sometimes weeks after admission, through simply waiting and watching the patient or by undertaking medical tests or surgery.

What these wards provide by way of career—which the emergency, ICU, or premature baby wards do not—is a place to take all the time necessary to die or to recover. The lingering trajectory is acceptable on these wards. The patient may stay on the ward for months or, if an "entry-reentry" patient, may go home and return several times during the course of his illness. Patients take all the dying time they need, and the staff provide the comforts needed while dying, a major one being painkillers. These wards provide time for continual, careful redefinitions of the dying trajectory, and the necessary treatments and attentions appropriate for each successive stage. These wards, in short, are custodians of the long, often indeterminant, ordeal of dying. From these wards the patient goes home or to the morgue. (See Chapters IV and V.)

A number of issues relate to the central question of these wards: Who shapes the patient's living while he is dying? How much control does the staff allow him or his family over what activities? To what degree can the staff prepare the patient and his family for his death? How often shall they send the patient home, or out for a drive? How long, if at all, should the patient's life be prolonged? How often and for how long can the family visit? How should the last days and hours of the patient's life be shaped? These issues bear on the sentimental order of the medical ward as well as on the organization of work, a sentimental order rather different from that found on the "quick-dying" wards. Much of the work is routine, and monotonous for dying patients. The routine also raises motivational and morale problems for staff. Nurses are confronted frequently with the helplessness of there being "nothing more to do" for the patient. Even if dying remains uncertain, the "challenge" of caring for the patient is often little more than just waiting to see if drugs or treatments work, while providing physical and psychological comforts. There is seldom the heroic challenge of the quick-dying wards. Indeed if a patient starts to die quickly and needs emergency measures, he may be sent to the ICU or surgery for heroic saving.

These undramatic challenges proffer low-demand medical experiences and relatively "passive" gratification. Because of the long
period of time spent with patients and their families, nurses on
these wards tend to develop strong involvements as the ordeal
proceeds. In order to prevent erosion of their composure, they
also become adept at avoiding dying patients and their families.
But they cannot entirely avoid the upsetting effects of waiting for
a patient to die. Unlike on the quick-dying wards, where the intense technical challenge and short patient careers constantly support the sentimental order, on medical wards the sentimental order
runs deep into involvement, helplessness, and monotony of work.
It is more vulnerable because it has more sensitive boundaries
without the continual support of intense short-term work. On these
wards, the staff is more often in a distressed state over coping
with dying patients, death, and their grieving families throughout
the longer trajectories.

When placement of the patient in the medical wards is based
on the initial definitions of a dying trajectory, those who are
judged certain to die, whether soon or not, are placed in the
"critical" wings or rooms of the ward. Patients whose mode of
dying is offensive—for example, they smell, groan, or are disfigured—may be segregated, sometimes in single rooms. This separation of dying patients from others allows the staff to keep control of the work and sentiments surrounding the dying and to
localize the death rate within the ward. Depending on their
stamina and wishes, nurses can then be assigned to either dying
or recovering patients. To be sure, some patients on the dying end
of the ward may recover and some on the recovering end begin
to die, but the general character of each part of the ward remains;
and work and distribution of patients to nurses can be controlled
accordingly. The arrangement affords optimal control over threats
to the sentimental order of the wards; fewer nurses (and "the
right ones") confront deaths, most of which are expected.

As we have remarked, formulating definitions of dying may
take time; these wards provide work and sentimental orders appropriate to keeping the staff accustomed to waiting days, weeks,

or sometimes even years for a presumably definitive diagnosis. While a patient's dying trajectory is indeterminant, they mark time, keeping him on the recovery end of the ward. Meanwhile, they tentatively consider a variety of possible trajectories. Often stories develop about the patient during this waiting period—a "fantasy" aspect to the sentimental order. Nurses have remarked on the "unreal" quality of waiting for clear indicators of the dying trajectory.

During the waiting, the patient may undergo tests or surgery. These procedures usually speed up the formulation of the trajectory. Tests may give useful answers in a few hours or ten days; surgery typically provides critical information before the sutures are in, or not at all. However, neither assures a conclusive diagnosis. The staff may have to return to waiting, to making educated guesses and theoretical interpretations, to developing a number of possible trajectories, and to seeking more tests and perhaps more surgery.

While the medical wards provide time for this waiting, the family and patient rarely join in the waiting. They want immediate answers: "What's wrong?" "What's going to happen?" The staff is forced to "string them along" while this temporal conflict lasts. For example, a woman entered one medical ward in a semicomatose state. The staff initially could find nothing wrong with her. They waited and watched for a week until she became conscious—still nothing. They decided to run blood tests—still nothing of special significance. Then they took her to surgery for a bone marrow biopsy, and found inconclusive evidence of leukemia cells. The doctors conferred, reviewing each symptom, but only came to a series of possible interpretations, no determinant type of dying trajectory.

As the waiting dragged on, it was increasingly stressful on the resident responsible for the patient. As he said, "Look, I've got these relatives here, and they want to know what's going to happen to her. Before I tell them that she's got leukemia and is going to die, I want to get a better specimen." The other doctors agreed, only half-expecting the resident to get more conclusive evidence.

They were content to continue waiting and "theorizing." But the resident, under pressure from the relatives, wanted to try another biopsy. "You just can't keep stringing people along this way," he argued. "It's been two weeks now, and each afternoon I have to give him [the son] some vague answer like, 'She's still in observation and we will know something more definite later.' If it was my mother, I would be anxious as hell to know what's going on." In the end the resident admitted he did not trust the pathologist, who himself was not sure of the leukemia cells, so he sent the patient home undiagnosed, and the waiting continued. Since leukemia is linked with an entry-reentry, lingering trajectory, they would find out soon enough if the patient were dying—probably on her next stay in the hospital.

This characteristic example shows the less dramatic, time-consuming dying trajectory on the medical wards. Even the challenge to the doctor to come up with accurate, subtle diagnosis is an ordeal compared to the adventure of the fast discovery of trajectories on the quick-dying wards. Similarly, the cure and recovery, even where possible, are often less technically sophisticated and heroic than in quick-dying wards; if not, the patient would be sent to the ICU.

AWARENESS OF INITIAL DEFINITIONS

Entering a hospital and being admitted to a ward entail a maze of social conditions and processes that give the various concerned persons varying states of awareness of the initial dying trajectory. These definitions become the basis of their ensuing behavior toward each other. These conditions and processes result in patient and family awareness of initial definitions, whether or not doctors decide to state them explicitly. (Most doctors hedge and do not clearly disclose "certain" dying.) They give rise to constant debate among the staff as to whether the patient "really knows" when he has not been told. They give rise also to awareness of the many dimensions of dying trajectories, such as certainty, duration, shape, mode, and so forth. Whether the resulting awareness is relatively accurate or inaccurate, these conditions and processes typically result in varying initial definitions of the dying trajectory. As a result, in the beginning of the hospital career, family, patient and staff tend easily to "talk past" each other, often doubting and distrusting each other's questions and avoiding giving answers. In this section we shall describe these various conditions and processes of admittance as they affect nurses, patients, and family.

Doctors and Nurses. The official initial definition of the dying trajectory is, as we have noted, made by the doctor in charge of the case. He either sends the patient to the hospital on the basis of this initial definition, or defines the trajectory when the patient enters the hospital and ward. Whether a doctor tells the nurses of a dying trajectory depends on several conditions. If there is plenty of time, the doctor may not tell them until later in the trajectory. But even in quick trajectories, he may not, for a variety of reasons, tell the nurses. He may see no need. One doctor—perhaps a bit more blunt than most—explained quite simply: "Why would we talk to the nurses?" He expected them to know through experience and viewing the patient's condition, and also on the basis of the patient's entry to the hospital. For example, he may have noted the trajectory on the patient's record or admittance forms, or put the patient on a critical list. The kind of treatments he prescribes may indicate his initial definition. Indeed, nurses may tell the doctor an initial definition—for example, by their alarm in coming to him after viewing an emergency patient. He also may not wish the nurses to know a patient is on the verge of dying in order to maintain their motivation to help him recover. Nurses may realize the patient is dying from the behavior of family "members" after they have been told by the doctor. Nurses also tell each other, depending on the most experienced among them for a reliable definition.[1]

Family and Patients. After the patient is admitted, it is typ-

1. See for our research on these problems of awareness *Awareness of Dying, op. cit.,* especially pp. 16–26.

ical for the doctor to make some kind of initial report to him and to his family. But seldom does he clearly indicate a dying trajectory at such an early stage of the hospital career. He usually gives vague reports to both, suggesting that it will take time for an adequate diagnosis; he thus gives himself time for later clarifications and redefinitions of the dying trajectory and of the potential hospital career of the patient. Temporal conflicts between staff and family and patients begin with these initial reports.

The major exception occurs in the case of imminent death, when it is important to tell the family in advance, so they can start preparing themselves immediately. In these situations, even if it is not advisable to tell a family member, procedures often give the true definition away. For example, the hospitalized mother who has delivered a preemie who may soon die is asked to sign admittance papers at any time, night or day; if the baby will probably live, there is time to ask her after breakfast. In some cases there is no time, and the family is told that the patient has died soon after admittance.

Typically, the doctor tells the patient the least of anyone, especially at admittance. His silence constrains the nurses also to silence—or evasions. However, so much happens at admittance that the patient, if conscious, has much to go on in establishing an initial illness trajectory, even if not quite able to describe it as a "dying" one.

Being sent to a hospital may in itself indicate to the patient, in several ways, that perhaps he is dying. He is sent at a moment's notice in an ambulance. He is sent to a medical center for special treatment instead of to the hospital where he formerly went. He is sent for unusual tests. He just wakes up in a hospital after an accident or stroke. Geriatric patients are sent to an age-segregated institution known to be the "end of the road," or knowing that "it is all over but the dying." At admission, it may be suggested that they sell their property. Or previous experience in hospitals may indicate to a patient that this is the "last trip."

The kind of ward to which the patient is admitted is sometimes a telling definition of his potential hospital career and trajectory. The quick-dying wards are immediately obvious to the patient, and he knows what it may mean to be rushed to emergency, the ICU, or the operating room. In some hospitals the medical wards are highly segregated, and the patient knows if he is placed on the cardiovascular, cancer, or geriatrics ward, for example. (In one cancer hospital in Japan we found a sign over the entrance designating this condition—an ample cue to the patient.)

However, even the patient who starts out on a general medical ward, where it is unlikely for him to guess his trajectory, can realize an initial dying trajectory if he is suddenly rushed to another ward, *e.g.,* the ICU. This is especially telling when the transfer occurs unannounced—"in order not to alarm" the patient! Instead, he may easily panic at the realization of why he is being transferred. This occurs with geriatric patients when transferred to a "death valley," an ICU designated to minister to their last days. In our terms, this transfer indicates that people are not likely to die quickly on the previous ward, and therefore his trajectory is no longer acceptable there. A patient may try to hide symptoms and pain from the staff in order to convince them that his condition is acceptable to the ward—a strategy that almost inevitably fails. The dread of transfer may lead patients to say to any staff member that happens by, "Don't let them transfer me." Not all patients, however, are aware enough to realize the meaning of a transfer.

Once on the ward, several things happen that also indicate to the patient the possibility of his dying. The treatments and tests ordered may serve as cues. It may be some personal reaction that informs him: one patient said about suspecting cancer, "It happened when I noticed that all the fun has gone out of eating," in spite of the reputation of the hospital's food. The kinds of patients on the ward and what is happening to them are also indicators of a possible dying trajectory. For example, one patient who woke up on an ICU complained about the noise and complaints of two patients across from him all night long. He said, "I'll bet they are dying." Immediately an initial definition of his own condition occurred to him.

The arrival of a priest is a sure sign. And when relatives come and start praying, appear anxious and fearful, come very often, try hard to conceal grave concern, continually assure the patient he will have the "best" treatment in this hospital, and so forth, it is again not hard to imagine what might be happening. A little girl said she thought she might die "because my mother and father are going to church all the time now."

The way the staff relates to the patient upon his admission may provide additional grounds for initial definitions of dying. They may seem very brusque and urgent in administering "heroic" or unusual treatments. They may withdraw when the patient asks what they are doing, creating the very suspicions they wish to prevent. When pinned down, the nurse may "pass the buck" to a doctor who cannot come because he is "too busy." Patients discover early in their hospital career that a dying patient tends to be avoided and his questions circumvented. Patients express feelings of being "trapped and helpless." Some actually telephone their families and ask to be taken home. They realize that the paucity of information given by staff at their entry to the hospital may well continue until they recover or die, unless they can find ways to overcome the barriers to awareness set up by staff and hospital organization.

Where and how a patient is placed on the ward upon admission or soon after can also be for him a very telling indicator of his chances for recovery, especially if he has had some experience in hospitals either as patient or visitor. For example, being placed in a room alone with the door left ajar, being screened off immediately after being placed in a multipatient room, or being placed as close to the nursing station as possible can lead to realizations that perhaps he is dying. These realizations are based both on comparisons with other patients, indicating that the common ward career does not entail isolation, and on the recognition that isolation prevents one's dying from disturbing other patients.

In short, the patient's trajectory is not quite acceptable, and he is being provided a slightly different career. Explaining to themselves the unusual placements may easily lead both patient and family to formulate definitions of a dying trajectory.

The definitions of a dying trajectory that may occur to a patient as he passes through the conditions and procedures of entering a hospital and ward are just beginning and concern mostly the certainty (or uncertainty) of dying. Definitions of time, mode and shape of trajectory come later. Whether or not correct, the initial definitions will be imbued with doubt, and are, therefore, liable to much redefinition as the patient's trajectory and hospital career proceed with their attendant changing conditions.

How a patient, a doctor, a nurse or a family member defines a dying trajectory becomes the basis for his or her behavior in connection with treating and handling the patient. In the remainder of this book, we shall discuss at length the changing definitions of the dying trajectory and the behavioral and interaction consequences of these changes at each stage of the trajectory.

IV

Lingering Trajectories: Institutional Dying

It does not take much reflection to see that what hospital staffs, as well as patients' families, commonly term "lingering deaths" comprise a rather varied class of trajectories with certain features in common. Both their differing and their common features affect the work and problems of hospital staffs when caring for lingering patients.

INSTITUTIONAL ORGANIZATION FOR SLOW DECLINE

In many countries, special institutional provision is made for people who are expected to live for some time while dying slowly. The United States has nursing homes and the geriatric wards typically found in state mental hospitals and in Veterans Administration and city or county hospitals. Some large cities, like New York, also have hospitals devoted almost exclusively to the care of elderly patients who are expected to die, frequently rather slowly, while in the hospital. (When tuberculosis was more often fatal, hospital staffs at TB hospitals also cared for many patients who died in visibly slow stages.) Many other countries have established similar kinds of institutions, whose chief, or at least one important, function is to free the dying patient's family from the task of caring for him during a potentially long physical decline. Sometimes, of course, the patient has no immediate family to care for him anyway.

THE PATIENTS

The typical patient in these institutions or on these wards has one or more known chronic diseases. Although patients are of various ages, they tend to be elderly; even those chronologically middle-aged or young are, so to speak, "physiologically aged" because of the character of their diseases. When sent to these institutions, they are not necessarily near death; they may only be so chronically ill as to suffer from permanently limited mobility, or so senile as to be unable to care for themselves.

Many are deposited at the site (often far from their home) by families who thereafter visit only infrequently. Other patients are quite literally abandoned to the establishment by kinfolk who wish to see no more of them, sometimes because they are considered so senile as to be no longer fully alive. In state mental hospitals, a characteristic route into the "old folks" wards leads from another ward when the patient has grown senile or incapable of caring for his own bodily necessities. Some of these patients sent from elsewhere in the hospital or from other hospitals in the state system have been there for many years, even decades; their families are no longer alive or are too far away to visit. These establishments succeed in sending relatively few patients back "into society." They do this only if a patient is sufficiently recovered to leave, or if the family desires or can be persuaded to take a manageable patient home. Both these conditions for leaving the establishment happen infrequently.

These locales vary considerably in the proportion of patients perceived as "dying," and there is also wide variation in how long a time passes between entry and death. At nursing homes and state hospitals, even on the geriatric services, patients may live for many years. On the other hand, some die shortly after entry.[1] Whether they die very slowly or relatively quickly, they tend to die during the inclement winter and summer seasons.

At any one time, a fair number of these patients may be comatose, and a large proportion of the rest are more or less senile. The physical decline to death is sometimes very gradual, with barely discernible passages into unmistakable senility, then into further reduced functioning ("going downhill mentally"), and finally into a comatose state. Even the more senile may live for many years. Of course, when a patient obviously near the end of his life is brought in, though he may linger a month or more, his downward course is more noticeable, as well as more noted by the staff. With these two kinds of expectable death—one faster, one slower, but both taking considerable time—there are a few surprise deaths. Occasionally a patient dies much sooner than the staff anticipated, as from a heart attack, but the event is quickly dismissed because it falls well within the overall range of what is expected for these patients. But, "most patients go down day by day and finally die, or they fall, break something, go to surgery and don't make it," and "most patients are comatose at the end."

WORK: ITS CONDITIONS AND ORGANIZATION

Except perhaps in private nursing homes for wealthy patients, these establishments for the hopelessly old, sick, and dying tend to have a low ratio of personnel per patient. Because the care is largely custodial, the bulk of the personnel is nonprofessional, with little or no specialized training other than what may be received on the job or through "in-service" education. In some state mental hospitals, "worker" patients, who are housed else-

1. For instance, at the state hospital we studied, geriatric patients were scattered throughout several chronic wards. Of a total of 1,825 patients more than 65 years of age, 65 had entered the hospital more than 20 years earlier, whereas 600 had been in the hospital less than two years. In the previous year, 175 patients of the 65+ group had died within a month of admittance. The hospital has from 30 to 60 geriatric deaths a month, with considerable fluctuation by season: during the winter and hot summer there are many more deaths.

where in the hospital, serve as supplementary personnel. Although the medical care given by physicians and registered nurses may be sophisticated and considerable, it is after all given to patients with long-term, chronic disorders and debilities—problems that ordinarily do not greatly excite the physician's interest or provide the nurse with the absorbing challenges or great rewards possible when there is a prospect of recovery. Neither the rate of pay nor the working conditions usually are such as to attract the best-trained, or at least the most ambitious, professionals, except in some county or city hospitals to which young interns and residents are drawn "for experience" and relative autonomy—but there, too, the terminal geriatric patients are among the least interesting cases for them.

This situation does not mean that these patients fail to receive good medical, nursing, or custodial care; they receive the type of care that the family or the state feels is merited in view of their advanced physical deterioration. Medical treatment and nursing care are aimed principally at slowing deterioration, thus prolonging life and keeping the patient reasonably comfortable during his last years, months, and days. Keeping him comfortable entails not only appropriate medication and sophisticated nursing, but the more ordinary custodial operations; the latter, indeed, bulk large in the daily work of the nurses and nursing assistants.

The presence of a considerable ratio of senile or comatose patients makes custodial work even more prominent than otherwise it might be. Numbers of those patients need to be kept clean; they must be taken to the toilet or serviced if they cannot manage the trip; they need to be fed, and perhaps even dressed. In short, whether or not most patients are explicitly perceived as dying, work must be organized to take care of a certain proportion of patients who are regarded by the staff as socially, if not biologically, dead.

When a patient is so sick as to be put on the "critical list," usually he is nearing his biological death as well. Extra staff time and effort is expended, although if the patient is judged hopelessly close to the end, usually only purely custodial work is done. These critical patients may be bedded down near the nursing station, rails may be put up to prevent their falling out of bed, and generally a closer eye is kept on their physical condition.

When the end approaches, little or no dramatic attempt is made to prolong life. These patients are believed to have "earned" their deaths because of their advanced age or extreme deterioration. So there are few "heroics"—last-ditch attempts to save lives —performed here. The prolonging of life consists, rather, of a steady daily effort. An appropriate metaphor to picture this effort is that of a conscientious staff braced on a hillside holding back a large rolling stone, which can only be slowed in its slow, inevitable fall to the bottom of the hill. An occasional reprieve, albeit temporary, adds to the staff's incentive to maintain life as long as it seems sensible to do so. There is a minimum of restiveness among personnel about keeping a patient alive when he "should be allowed to die," for consensus is relatively high about letting the flickering spark disappear when "the time has come." But there are exceptions. As a nurse at a state hospital said: "I'm not alone, but I am in the minority on saving lives. I'll put them on penicillin, and they'll say 'Why?' We *are* causing some discomfort when we keep them alive like this, so I can see their point."

So, unlike dying patients in other types of medical facilities, who may present crises for the staff, these dying patients present few. Crisis may arise from other sources, however, as when increased workloads are brought about by unexpected turnover among the staff or by seasonal peaks in the death rate. (One nurse we interviewed at a state hospital had lost considerable weight during a recent seasonal peak.) Changes in state and VA hospital policies or functions may critically affect their geriatric wards. VA hospitals are now experiencing a complex instance of the latter type of change: a steady rise in numbers of aged and terminal patients is altering the character of these hospitals all over the nation.

MANAGEMENT OF THE DYING TRAJECTORY

Medical and custodial management of the dying patient is one thing, but what about the management of the patient's day-in, day-out behavior during his lingering dying? And what of the responses of his family, of other patients, and of the personnel themselves?

We can begin to answer those questions by emphasizing that these institutions have a kind of slow-moving, timeless quality; after all, they are set up to care for patients who may linger for months or years. The chief rationale that sustains both the personnel and such families as do visit is that these patients "deserve" to die; indeed, as we have mentioned, they often are regarded as socially dead before their actual biological deaths ("My dad died the day he got this way").

But the staff makes fine distinctions among the patients under their care; there are degrees of senility. There are also degrees of likeability; staff members can easily get attached to these old people if they are not entirely senile. When they finally die, the staff may experience sadness, missing "the old fellow." On the whole, however, a complex interlacing of personal trajectories (such as we shall note in later chapters) is noticeably missing. Both personnel and family are effectively protected against a sense of deep loss by their judgments that these patients' lives no longer have much value to themselves, to their families, or to the larger society: "He was so old." "He'd lived a long life." "It's better really that he died, he's better off." "Naturally you hate to see them go—but old people I don't mind seeing go so much as younger." "You feel both ways; some you're attached to and so you feel badly, but they're 80 or 90 and I figure. . . ." Thus are the deaths written off.

The patient himself may have little control over management of his dying, especially during its later phases. If he becomes senile before his dying becomes obvious to him, he offers no alternatives to the staff's shaping of his trajectory. If not senile, he is likely to have come to terms with his own eventual or relatively immediate dying. ("Some actually verbalize they want to die. They've lived their span of life. They're 'no more good in the world.'") Even if a patient has not come to clear terms with the prospect of death, typically he is unlikely to bother the personnel with his forebodings or personal grievings. Personnel report few attempts by patients to broach such subjects: "Patients don't talk of dying. I did have one patient recently who asked if she were dying—but she doesn't remember it now."

On the other hand, as a nurse in a Scottish hospital said, elderly patients may indicate acceptance of death and although they "don't talk about it with us, among themselves they talk about buying burial grounds or having made preparations." These rehearsals of death are not necessarily shared with the staff, who, the patients feel, simply may not understand. (As one elderly ex-patient from a metropolitan hospital told us, "The staff just didn't understand why so many of those patients wanted to die.") As we recorded in *Awareness of Dying*,[2] in one hospital for patients "at the end of the road," where the average duration of dying was only six months, mutual pretense about dying was almost universal between patients and staff: neither raised the issue of death. Geriatric wards at city and county hospitals also tend to engage in this type of pretense. All these attitudes mean that the staffs have relatively good control—usually considered desirable in itself—managing dying trajectories.

This management is little interfered with by either families or other patients. The families are unlikely to be around much, if at all, during the last days and hours of life. If near geographically, they have still tended, because of the lingering character of dying, to fall away, reducing the number of their visits, perhaps asking on the phone, "Is he any better today?" or inquiring if it is worthwhile coming today, or if he can recognize them today. Even those who have previously been attentive may drift away. As they see it, there is nothing more that they can do.

2. *Op. cit.*, p. 64.

Other patients may be unaware that someone has become critically ill or has died; if aware, they may give little or no indication of concern. If depressed by the actual death, they are unlikely to discuss the matter with the personnel—while the personnel are equally unlikely to discuss it with the patients. This general silence is all the more striking because in some geriatric wards the dying patient is visible to everyone; in others, moving the patient and his bed elsewhere clearly signifies "dying." As one technician remarked, "The ones who are alert . . . if a patient is sick they know, just like we do, that he'll either get better or not. If a patient dies, sometimes the others are upset but sometimes they don't even know." His associate added, "Occasionally one of the better patients will ask, 'Did she die?' I say yes, but there is very little stir on this type of ward." And another technician: "Some of the better patients will ask sometimes about whether someone died, but there is never any discussion really. Some have said, 'She's better off.' " In short, brief snatches of open awareness may occur, but mostly there is closed, or mutual-pretense awareness between patients and staff. All this contributes to the staff's shaping of a dying patient's dying trajectory.

The actual death tends to be quite uneventful, for "they lie crippled . . . like a shell and sometimes we even almost forget them" except for popping in and "giving a little physical care." (That was the description given by a nurse in a Scottish hospital, but American personnel make equivalent statements about these deaths.) Post-mortem "scenes" with grieving families, so characteristic of other kinds of deaths, are here almost totally lacking. Families may not appear at all; they no longer exist, or they have abandoned their kinsman, or they live too far away to get to the hospital quickly, if at all. The institution is geared, however, for processing the family through a post-mortem routine. If a family appears, it is informed of the death; responsible members sign papers, may be asked about an autopsy, are given valuables. Sometimes funeral arrangements have long since been marked in the patient's chart or "sometimes when we wire the relatives or phone we will ask about them." And sometimes "we ask them to wire about the autopsy." If hospital records show no relatives, or if known kin do not respond to the announcement of death, standard burial or cremation arrangements are made with local authorities. In any event, these relatives are far less likely to "break down" than are those who are confronted with more traumatic types of death. ("I think the day they brought them here was the day they gave them up. That is worse than the dying—for them and for us.")

Sentimental Order and Its Disturbance

In effect, then, these patients drift out of the world, sometimes almost like imperceptibly melting snowflakes. The organization of work emphasizes comfort care and custodial routine, and is complemented by a sentimental order emphasizing patience and inevitability. The sentimental order is disrupted or shattered from time to time by events associated with a patient's dying. These events fall principally into three classes involving mode of dying, relatives' nonacceptance of the dying or of the death itself, and reactions of other patients.

Mode of dying rarely produces visibly disruptive effects. But, as a Scottish nurse noted, one strain on her was "the wasting away into a skeleton of some patients." It is hard to say how much strain less self-aware staff members actually endure; however, the slow decline of a patient does not precipitate many visibly shocked responses among the staff. Other patients' reactions are also minimally disturbing to the sentimental order of the establishment. The main danger stems from the reactions of family members, either through direct disturbance of work itself or through more indirect changes of collective mood. In the Edinburgh hospital, for example, although a young man visited his dying mother only infrequently, he added to their work since the staff rather than he was then responsible for laundering her clothes; he only took them home when he visited. This made them very resentful of the young man. As another elderly Scottish patient lay dying, her daughter "never could understand . . . after all, the lady was 94." The daughter raised an unusual commotion right through the post-mortem period. In short, unpredictable family reactions can disturb the staff and interfere with its work.

Things occasionally go awry in other ways, too:

> One time a wife and daughter spent the whole night. In the morning they were still there, and I couldn't get my patients up and dressed with them there very well—they weren't very good patients—naked and smelly, some of them—so I asked my supervisor if I couldn't get rid of them for an hour so I could get my patients up and cleaned. She said yes, and I asked them to leave. You could see the relief on their faces; I had *made* them go. I suggested they go into town for breakfast, which they did.

Or there may be a problem during the post-mortem process. For instance, the woman in charge of much of one hospital's post-mortem paperwork said:

> I've had a lot of letters recently from two Catholic sisters of a patient who died without any funds. They wrote saying they had no money for burial, so we cremated. Then they found out that a Catholic cemetery wouldn't accept ashes and they were furious. So I asked Father O'Hara to write them, and it's finally being straightened out because the cemetery will bury if they didn't authorize the cremation.

And sometimes relatives will visit shortly after a patient has died, not having yet received the hospital's telegraph announcement of the death. Either they left home too soon or there was some slip-up in the administrative machinery, such as the physician's tardy signing of the death certificate.

Sentimental order is more likely to be shattered by unexpected departures from the typical lingering trajectory. In the

Scottish geriatric hospital, the death from cancer of a 50-year-old patient (brought there because of his fatal disease) greatly affected the nurses. In an American nursing home, a sudden heart attack upset the staff. In a state hospital, a "patient worker" died unexpectedly and suddenly, so that "even the patients were upset." Of course, work order and sentimental order can be disrupted by conditions of work that have nothing to do with dying patients, but that is quite another issue.

As we have intimated earlier, the satisfactions of working with lingering patients derive in part from the relatively stable sentimental orders of establishments caring for them. Life there is relatively unruffled, in comparison with most medical hospitals. The relative absence of visiting family members and the relative passivity of patients contribute to a regularity of routine; so does the relative expectability of the dying trajectories. Personnel manage to keep fair control over the shaping of those trajectories. Although the outsider may think the atmosphere of these places depressing, the personnel take pleasure in keeping these patients comfortable and, if possible, alive. Their satisfactions are closely associated with having come to terms with "comfort care"—not undervaluing it by making comparisons with what others might consider "real" medical and nursing "cure" care.

Like these institutions themselves, the personnel are rather well adjusted—except during occasional crises that disrupt work and sentimental orders—to cope with any and all phases of slow dying; no matter how slow the dying and no matter how blurred the boundaries of the phases. Indeed, this is a chief feature of these institutions.

IDEOLOGY AND INSTITUTIONALIZED DYING

The general patterns evinced by most locales specifically for geriatric and other deteriorated patients are altered somewhat in those rare institutions where special ideologies guide terminal care. Among the best known is St. Joseph's Hospice in London, about which Dr. Cicely Saunders has written extensively.[3] Dr. Saunders worked out, at this hospital, her ideology and its associated operational philosophy of terminal care.[4] The heart of her rationale is that St. Joseph's, as a "specialized unit" for terminal patients, "does not have the challenge of diagnoses nor the difficult decisions concerning treatment . . . those stages of their illnesses are now over."[5]

It follows that staff are to look at these incurable patients (virtually all at St. Joseph's are incurable) as "persons in distress" and to "concentrate on giving them relief."[6] Relief—in our terms, comfort care—consists of several elements. First of all, since "at this stage of illness, pain is nearly always continuous," a program of "continuous control is called for." (Dr. Saunders has written in some detail about the pharmacological aspects of her program.) A most important dictum is that "drugs must be given regularly" and no patient kept waiting in fear or anxiety "until the 'proper' time."[7] Dr. Saunders emphasizes the importance not only of carefully tailored pain control itself, but also of establishing and maintaining the patient's trust in the staff's ability to keep him reasonably free from pain, until death if necessary. The philosophy is that the "care of the dying demands all that we can do to enable patients to *live* until they die . . . and includes the care of the family, the mind, and the spirit as well as the care of the body."[8] Consequently, the establishment of the patient's trust involves the willingness to openly discuss dying with him if he himself recognizes he is dying and chooses to embark on that

3. "The Last Stages of Life," *American Journal of Nursing,* Vol. 65 (March, 1965); "Care of the Dying," *Nursing Times* reprint (London: Macmillan, 1959); "The Need for Institutional Care for the Patient with Advanced Cancer" (paper written for the Cancer Institute, Madras); *Care of the Dying* (London: Macmillan, 1960); "The Symptomatic Treatment of Incurable Malignant Disease," *Prescribers' Journal,* Vol. 4 (1964), pp. 68–74.

4. For a distinction between those terms, see Anselm Strauss *et al.,* *Psychiatric Ideologies and Institutions* (New York: Free Press of Glencoe, 1965), pp. 8, 360.

5. C. Saunders, "The Last Stages of Life," *op. cit.,* p. 1.

6. *Ibid.*

7. *Ibid.,* pp. 2–3.

8. *Ibid.,* p. 2.

topic, as well as the obligation to respond appropriately to indirect and even nonverbal approaches to the topic. In any event, staff response to a patient is to be guided by the situation, allowing him to "come to the insight in his own way and time." Above all, their responses must reflect due regard for the patient's own requirements and his dignity. The objective is to help "mobilize the patient's own resources" and allow him to "come to his own personal victory." [9] Dr. Saunders offers convincing evidence that this philosophy works with many patients, and notes that they "have handed on strength and confidence to the others and to all who had the privilege of knowing them." [10]

Of the structural conditions under which dying takes place at St. Joseph's, the following points seem clear: Of a total of 150 beds, "forty to fifty are kept for patients with terminal malignant disease who are sent by other hospitals or by family physicians with a prognosis of three months or less; only 10 per cent live longer than that time. The remaining beds . . . are for the frail with no homes and for patients with long-term illness who are not suited for more active units, not for patients needing rehabilitation." [11] Patients are housed in six-bed units. Nursing personnel are not given unusual training (there are also nuns at this hospital). Patients are not moved to separate rooms when near death.

All in all, St. Joseph's is a last stage, comfort-care hospital, not notably different from the Scottish one discussed above. A main difference, however, is that all terminal patients are dying from malignant disease. Hence the ideology of keeping patients free from pain and helping them achieve a corresponding freedom from fear by sustaining open awareness when needed is highly relevant to shaping these lingering trajectories.

The staff's basic strategy involves shaping each trajectory in conjunction with the patient's own conceptions of how it should be shaped. Primary in cancer is the fear—sometimes all too justified—of dying in constantly severe pain. An important aspect

9. *Ibid.*
10. *Ibid.*, p. 4.
11. *Ibid.*, p. 2.

of the patient's conception of his trajectory is that there be no pain. If this is medically possible, the staff promise him permanent relief, build his trust in their capacity to carry out that promise, and point to the patients who are further along in dying (or who may already have died) as examples of their ability to control pain. The patients' stories are the staff's "success stories"; the staff can point to many such stories.

Another key structural element in this hospital is the personal activity of Dr. Saunders, both as a reliever of pain and as a psychologist who sustains her patients. The latter role is called for especially when patients are aware of their own nearing demise, as most at this hospital are. Patients' awareness relates, in turn, to the staff's ability to "deliver." They are able to help the patient lose his undue anxiety about dying itself and come to terms with his past life, if need be, precisely because he *is* cognizant of his dying. It is also important for the patient to have sufficient time to come to terms with his imminent death; quick death might leave him dying in psychological agony and with many unresolved life problems, whereas a lingering dying without pain helps establish his trust in the staff by providing "proof."

Another important condition for the effective operation of the sustaining ideology is, as we shall see more fully later, the absence of families or the presence of only fully cooperative ones. Without this condition, difficulties are encountered. As Dr. Saunders notes apropos of what we have termed "open" and "closed" awareness:

> Relatives vary as patients do in their desire for the truth and many ask that the patient should not be told and prefer to try to keep up normal relationships. Some do this successfully to the end. Others may need to be restrained from over-acting or helped to see when the patient really wants to be honest with them. One patient was greatly distressed because as she gradually realized she was dying her husband remained apparently cheerful and oblivious.

However, the guiding philosophy of the staff enabled them to tell this husband "what was happening and [he] was able at last to show her how much he cared." [12]

That the sentimental order may also be disrupted by patients who respond negatively or not at all to the prevailing ideology is suggested by the case of a patient noted as "difficult to help." [13] This unmarried, middle-aged German expatriate was a very isolated and withdrawn person, despite her fair knowledge of English. "Her mental suffering was all too apparent. She was extremely difficult to help and comfort because her whole experience and personality made such an illness and the publicity of a general ward well nigh intolerable to her. The nursing staff found her difficult to handle and she found them hard to understand." She repeatedly refused medicines. She complained that the staff was doing nothing for her or "were making her worse by what we gave her." She also "clutched so hard at any sign of improvement that it seemed wrong to be frank with her." In short, she played havoc with the sentimental order, if not with the work order itself. The situation was saved, almost miraculously, when Dr. Saunders asked a German friend, a trained psychiatric nurse, to talk with the patient. Although the patient died without awareness of her dying, the psychiatric nurse was able to talk sufficiently deeply with her to get her to express various fears and troubles, so that the patient "seemed comforted and peaceful at last" before becoming comatose and quickly dying.

Two additional structural conditions apparently exist in the wards under Dr. Saunders' direction. Each condition is crucial for the success of terminal care there. One has been implied in discussing the "difficult case": a patient must willingly delegate his care to the staff. As we shall see later, some patients in all countries, and many patients in some countries, do not delegate care to professionals when near death. In fact, it is useful to draw a distinction between the willingness to delegate partial control to the hospital and the willingness to delegate virtually total control.

12. C. Saunders, *Care of the Dying, op. cit.,* p. 8.
13. *Ibid.,* pp. 16–18.

The difficult woman discussed above was willing to go to the hospital but made plain by various actions, some highly dramatic (*e.g.,* bursting into tears at one point and complaining about English doctors), that she was not ceding much control over her life to the hospital staff. The other structural condition is that St. Joseph's can function so capably with terminal patients precisely because its staff is able to fulfill promises about keeping pain under control. Patients in Asian or African countries, where drugs tend to be both scarce and expensive, cannot always be promised freedom from their pain. This single structural difference—the relative availability of pain-control drugs—would make a crucial difference in the interaction between the staff and the patients under their care.

One final point: at St. Joseph's, the satisfactions that patients and staff derive from their joint management of the lingering trajectory are undeniable. If such management works well, pain and anxiety are minimized, while acceptance of death is maximized. The patient can live with dignity and even some pleasure while dying gracefully. Staff need not cope with unpleasant "scenes" and are able to take satisfaction in contributing to courageous and relatively peaceful deaths. For Dr. Saunders and the institution, each "success story" contributes to strengthening the ideology, and often also adds to medicine's knowledge of pain control in terminal cancer cases.

REHEARSALS AND INSTITUTIONALIZED DYING

In America, tuberculosis used to be a dreaded, often fatal, disease. Nowadays, few Americans die in hospitals from tuberculosis; most patients eventually leave for home. In Greece, a 10-year-old TB hospital that we visited also showed the impact of the new treatments. Only 100 of its 200 beds were in use, for mainly older patients. In this kind of specialty hospital, the staff gives care to patients who have the same disease but are at different stages of getting better or worse. Of course, every patient knows he has tuberculosis, and each understands that anyone who dies from it almost invariably suffers a slow decline.

This knowledge, combined with the relative slowness of change for better or worse, results in a continual search by each patient for signs of his own "movement." [14] Signs of worsening are quite visible, so that if a patient discovers that he is losing considerable weight or spitting blood, he cannot escape being aware of his worsening condition. Moreover, since every patient has the same disease, one who is worsening is likely to have a visible model before his eyes. Quite literally, by viewing other patients he can rehearse his own fate, usually more than once. In consequence, this kind of hospital is distinguished by considerable depression and agitation among a number of patients.

At the Greek hospital we visited, these reactions were a great problem for the staff. Patients showed by visible gesture their fears of decline, and "lost courage" when they saw signs of their own deterioration in others. (One elderly patient, "to attract attention," as a staff member explained, would from time to time claim that he was dying, showing fright at the prospect.) The staff had, by its own admission, few effective tactics with which to counter the pessimistic rehearsals of dying patients. Neither could they do much to counteract the involvement of healthier patients with the dying, for what is visible to the dying person is equally visible to other patients. (Without mentioning why, healthier patients continually urged one dying patient to eat more.)

Staff problems are rendered all the more complex because, even though most patients are improving, they are not necessarily happy about the progress they perceive. They may be upset because they are not progressing faster. Or they may be angry at the staff because it assesses their rate of progress as slower than they believe it is, and limit their privileges accordingly.[15] While

14. Julius Roth has given a detailed description and analysis of this search and its consequences for hospitalized American patients, who seem now invariably to get better, in some degree. See his *Timetables* (Indianapolis: Bobbs-Merrill, 1963).

15. *Ibid.*, especially Chapter 3, "Conflict and Bargaining over the Timetable," pp. 30–59.

these individual and collective moods are a part of the daily tex-
ture of hospital life, the sentimental order, of course, is really
shattered by the occasional suicides of patients who have chosen
to shape their own dying trajectories—hastening death rather than
inching toward it as others, whom they have watched, have done.

It does not take much imagination to think metaphorically of
the staff as moving through a thick fog of patients' fantasies,
ranging from exultant and optimistic through pessimistic and
deeply despondent. One would think that under these circumstances there might be a fair amount of open talk about death.
However, at least between staff and patients, there seems not to
be, either about actual dying or about recent deaths. Mutual pretense prevails. Relationships between staff and patients are also
affected by the general lack of visiting by families. They visit infrequently because specialty hospitals tend to draw patients from
considerable distances away.

In the Greek hospital, patients came from villages so distant
that their kinsmen visited either not at all or only infrequently,
perhaps only when called just before the death. Moreover, tuberculosis is still considered by Greek peasants to be a stigmatizing
disease, a disgrace. Like mental or senile patients, tuberculosis
patients sometimes are abandoned by their families. The shame is
so great that a patient who gets well sometimes does not return
to his village, but seeks lodging and work in another village where
he can hide his tubercular past. If he returns home, and the family knows where he has been, it often maintains a fictional story
explaining his absence. In some cases, families are so ashamed of
their dying kinsman that they allow him to die unvisited, and
even fail to claim his body after death. This abandonment is all the
more striking because in other illnesses Greek families frequently
insist on taking a dying kinsman from the hospital so that he can
die at home. Understandably enough, abandoned patients display
anger at their families—anger that spills over to the staff and
affects patient-staff relationships.

Overall, then, dying in such a TB hospital is marked by the
following characteristics: Open awareness prevails, both about

the disease each patient has and about the fact that each patient is dying. All patients know when a colleague is dying (if he dies in the usual lingering way), and the dying patient knows it too and is likely to refer openly to it. Because signs of deterioration are so visible, and so well known by the patients, each dying patient is apt to have rehearsed his own death by watching others in their slow decline. The probability of at least one rehearsal is enhanced because tubercular dying usually is a slow process; the dying patient has had ample time in which to observe the last stages of another patient's dying trajectory. Rehearsal generally, and perhaps also the observed mode of dying, results in occasional suicides—the patient insists on managing how his trajectory will end. And because the families also have stigmatized views of what a tubercular trajectory is, or means, they often seem willing to declare their kinsmen socially, if not biologically, dead when he is committed to the hospital.

V

Lingering Trajectories: At Home and in Hospitals

In Chapter IV, we discussed how lingering trajectories are conceived and managed within special types of institutions or on special wards. While the TB hospital is not an end-of-the-road institution in the same sense as the geriatric hospital or the nursing home, it has rather obviously a connotation of finality for TB patients in countries where deaths from tuberculosis still occur relatively frequently. The same can be said for the medical wards of city and VA hospitals, where there are many elderly dying patients.

In contrast, the modern general hospital, with its corps of professionals, their numerous "paramedical" assistants, and its amazingly effective medical technology, is the epitome of a life-saving institution. This image is a product only of recent decades; general hospitals, too, used to be places where "you go to die." In countries less economically developed than the United States, this is how most people still regard their hospitals—and they do so realistically, since only the seriously ill are sent there. But in the United States and Western Europe, at least, hospitals have won such victories over illness as to counteract successfully, if not erase entirely, the old image of the "death house." Hospital staffs themselves perhaps take success so much for granted and are so little inclined to dwell on inevitable defeats (not all wards have deaths anyhow) that it takes occasional traumatic deaths to remind them that the hospital is not only a place where people *happen* to die, but also where they *come* to die and are *sent* to die. This is particularly true when the dying trajectory is expected to be a slow, lingering one.

DYING AT HOME

Some light can be shed on lingering trajectories in the hospital by first considering briefly what dying at home is like—whether or not the family finally yields its kinsman, or he yields himself, to the hospital during his last hours or days. Our data are drawn from interviews with nurses assigned by a public health agency to visit the homes of lower-income patients. Each nurse visited a number of patients; most were not regarded as "terminal cases," but typically had the degenerative diseases of old age.

Since most of these patients die at home rather than in a hospital or nursing home, a salient feature is their own or their family's wish to manage the dying for themselves. They do this, of course, with the help of the physician, who prescribes treatment and orders regimens, and with the additional good offices of the visiting nurse (or nurses) assigned from the public health agency. The most obvious problems of management—of caring for the patient—involve his physical needs. The closer he comes to death, usually the less he can do for himself. He must be bathed, shaved, have his pajamas changed, given the proper diet, and perhaps fed, given enemas, or watched for bedsores. Some of these operations are natural to ordinary family life, but some are not. Patients in great pain have to be bathed in special ways, for instance, and catheters have to be properly handled.

His wife really needed somebody; she was almost at her wit's end. He had so many bedsores. The day I went in was the first he hadn't been able to be helped to the bathroom. In just two days she and I had developed good teamwork. I'd lift, she'd put the bedpan under, and so on. He had two tubes that had to be drained (he had cancer of the bladder), and she was already doing that, but I taught her about other things, especially bedsore care, and gave her help on his diet, told her of things very sick people are more apt to eat—custard instead of oatmeal.

Since the nurse visits only occasionally, and the family supplies the steady workers, the nurse's teaching aims both to increase the patient's comfort and to ease the family's work. It also tries to ease family anxiety about the work. ("I like to stay long enough to really *explain* the care. If you just tell them what to do, sometimes you come back and find the patient in worse condition than you left him.") The nurse tends to coach family members about psychological matters. She may remind a wife not to whisper about her husband's condition when in his room, for he may still be capable of hearing. ("The wife whispered right around him, thinking he didn't hear. Even people who didn't have cancer would think they did with her around!") Or she may caution relatives not to treat the patient "like a baby."

When the nurse is first assigned to the patient, she may not even know that he is considered terminal; his physician may not have signified this. But if she knows, or becomes aware, then she is in a better position to anticipate what the patient and his family are up against as he nears death. The lay images of what will transpire are likely to be far less accurate than hers. If the family does not realize their kinsman is dying, then "you work it so they know it's terminal by the end . . . sort of drop hints on the way," or persuade the physician to tell the family.

The sooner the family members know something of what to expect, the better they can carry on between the nurse's intermittent visits. As one nurse complained:

> So often we don't get in on terminal cases until close to the end. It would be much better to start when they are still in the hospital. . . . It's so much better if, before the family faces the pressure and emotion of the patient home from the hospital, I can tell them about the disease, and what they will be able to do to work with us.

She concluded her remarks with, "They need more preparation when they know it's going to be a long thing, chronic or terminal." So, to some extent, the nurse coaches responsible family members about what to expect in the way of bodily deterioration and worsening symptoms, and the change of work that probably will be entailed by the patient's decline: "We talk to them about the nature of the disease and what to expect and how to take care of it. You fear things when you don't know about them, so knowledge of what to expect in a disease helps lower their anxiety." It is important also that they know something of what to expect because "sometimes a difficult thing is for us to get the person who is caring for the patient to do everything they ought to. They find it offensive, I guess." As the end draws near, the nurse may even step in and "question wives as to whether their husbands have drawn a will. . . . I've gotten the conversation along those lines, and then said I thought *everybody* should have a will—did her husband?" Whether or not she provides the family members with clear images of the anticipated trajectory, the nurse stands ready to signal them or answer their questions about what is happening right now, during the present phase of dying.

Several obstacles can frustrate the nurse in her efforts to coach family members in giving proper care to their patient. Sometimes they just do not understand the procedures, and she has to demonstrate them repeatedly. Sometimes kinfolk are recalcitrant —they know perfectly well how to care for the patient, and no outsider is going to show them. ("There's a problem in home nursing. In the hospital you are the boss. But at home you aren't the real voice of authority. Relatives will have ideas about diet, and they are on top, not you. Or home remedies.") The nurse may have to ask the physician to speak with more effective authority, though he will not always do so. Sometimes, as suggested earlier, the relative cannot face "offensive" aspects of the care (bad odors, for instance) and so cannot give proper nursing. The nurse may then attempt to counter possible guilt feelings: "Let them talk it out and reassure them there is reason for these feelings and that they are not alone in them."

There are also interpersonal relationships within families that decrease the efficiency of care. Perhaps the families serviced by the nurses we interviewed were even more prone to interpersonal difficulties than most, because many were only segments (or remnants) of families: an aged couple with no children; two sisters; a male patient and his two sisters-in-law who had come four years earlier to nurse him, and so on. ("The sister-in-law who took care of the housekeeping hated him and he knew it. . . . She said if only she had enough money she would leave. . . . She refused to help him; when he got very ill she wouldn't help with the bedpan, so we had to arrange things around him so he could help himself the best he could. . . . I always felt sorry for him, dying amid all that hostility.") Interpersonal family relations are extremely important to good comfort care, and nurses tend quickly to assess the prevailing temper of the household. They will judge a patient to be good, but his wife to be "difficult," or say that the attending husband is compassionate, thoughtful, and responsible, but that his wife is not at all a nice person. In this calculus of judgment, a cooperative family becomes increasingly necessary as the patient becomes less able to care for himself.

In the typical lingering death at home, the closer to the end, the more difficult the care becomes for the family members. The amount of deterioration and the work it entails are not easy for them to imagine unless they have experienced such deaths previously. Consequently, the nurse almost inevitably finds herself stepping up the number of her visits during this phase of dying: "Toward the end you generally have to start going in more frequently, and this gives you an idea the end is near." The nurse not only gives more physical care, but is likely to move in more on the family—sending them upstairs to rest, listening to their grieving, reassuring them about guilt over wishing the ordeal was over.

It is during precisely this period that some families get frightened, and cannot stand the pressure. (As one nurse said, "In general, if they die at home, it is very traumatic—they need 24-hour care and families can't do it. There are exceptions, of course.") Some families give in to the advice of the nurse or physician and let the patient go to the hospital or a nursing home. (Occasionally a patient has already been in a nursing home, but has been brought home because conditions there were distressing to him.) In general, however, the particular population visited by these agency nurses preferred to have its relatives die at home, possibly because of cost but also possibly, as one nurse suggested, because this older generation, holding older attitudes, still considers that hospitals are not good places in which to die.

Usually the visiting nurse is not present when the lingering patient dies at home. She may not know about the death until informed by phone. (One nurse remarked that she had once arrived at a house, on a "routine" visit, during the funeral.) But, by chance, the nurse sometimes plays some role in the painful last moments.

> Just once I was there when a patient died. She was my own age, and I was very attached to her. Her mother called me at home early in the morning and asked if I could come out. I told her I'd rearrange my schedule and visit them first. When I got there I saw that she was dying, so I called her mother in to hold her hand and then phoned the doctor. You must handle it as naturally as possible. I let her stay holding her hand until the doctor got there; it seemed to help her.

Nurses report that they visit the survivors during the post-mortem period, partly because their own personal careers have become "involved" and partly because, as nurses, they wish to help further. The family member may even request the nurse to return: "She asked me when we were on the phone at the time of her mother's death—she'd died the afternoon I went and found her failing—to please come back and see her—had made me promise. So I went and she told me all about the death." Or the nurse may casually visit once again just to see how things are: "I was in the neighborhood on a call about a week after the funeral and had a little spare time so I went to see her. And believe it or not, she was just as perky as could be! . . . She talked very calmly, wept a little, but not breaking down at all. Her children had asked her to sell her house and live with first one and then the other, but she said she wasn't going to do it." And the nurse's personal interest may be so great that she picks up news about the survivors much later; the nurse quoted directly above closed her narrative: "According to the RN in that neighborhood, who saw her recently, she has gained weight and looks well. . . . She must be 88 years old!"

Thus far we have emphasized three salient features in our account of lingering dying at home: first, the desire of the family and/or patient to shape the dying trajectory; second, the inter-relationships of the experiential careers of nurse and responsible kin, and how together they handle the care of the dying; and third, the importance of the mode of dying in determining whether the family can sustain the drama until its very end. The intersection of the personal careers of the nurse and the family members can also be an important feature of dying at home. If the nurse arrives early enough in the trajectory and visits frequently enough, she can become "personally involved." Since some patients are visited over as long a period as two or three years, involvement is quite understandable; but even much shorter periods can bring con-siderable emotional engagement. Nurse and patient get to like and trust one another. The nurse also may be drawn into family feuds, or find herself balancing carefully to stay "neutral."

While the engagement of visiting agency nurses with fam-ilies is probably not as great as that of private duty nurses, it is possible that the visiting nurse's involvement more directly affects the patient care, for since she must delegate most nursing care to the family members, their trust and their capacity to learn and follow through on instructions depends to a considerable degree on "personal" relationships with her. Some hazards of these in-volvements are suggested by these remarks:

I think you've got to try very hard to keep objective be-cause you're going to get a little emotionally involved any-way. The RN-patient relationship is better if you're not too close. They may get too dependent on one person and then another may have to take over. It shows even on the level of getting very upset if you don't come until two. You have to remind them that they have to be flexible—have to

> keep it on a professional level. . . . I know one nurse . . .
> she's in some sort of trouble with her supervisor because
> they started calling her instead of the department.

This nurse's most important point is the first: A nurse must balance her relationships among the various members of the family, and keep her eye on the main job—care of the patient. The linkage between getting "drawn in" and giving good nursing care is underlined, again, by the comment of another nurse that she makes "a conscious effort to stay somewhat aloof" because being too empathetic takes its toll on her. But "of course, you have to get somewhat involved—or else you seem a cold fish to the family. They have to feel you're interested, not just a do-gooder. It's a strange paradox." Another nurse confessed that "there's a tendency to become too involved. If you sense this, you just have to tell yourself: now's the time to watch out. . . . You can get so involved that you forget what you're basically there for." Her supervisor repeatedly tells her "not to get so involved."

Although the intersection of a nurse's personal career with those of the family entails hazards, deep satisfactions sometimes accrue to her. Those satisfactions include enhancement of self as well as pride in jobs well done. Presumably the family's chief satisfactions in managing to care for their relative while he dies at home turn around maintenance of family solidarity and fulfillment of proper obligations to the dying person. Whether family members are able to endure until the very end, it must be emphasized, is closely linked with mode of dying. The point is dramatically underscored by a story told us, ten years after the event, by a hospital nurse: Late at night her hospital received a frantic call from a family who had been taking care of a relative without any assistance from a nurse. Their patient obviously was dying, was "turning black," and they had been unable to reach a doctor. The hospital quickly assigned this nurse to visit the family. On her arrival, she found them all so distraught that she "had five patients on my hands." The experience convinced her that no patient should die outside a hospital. Under ordinary circumstances, when the family faces such an impossible emergency, the patient is sent to the hospital rather than the hospital to the patient.

LINGERING OUTSIDE, BUT QUICK DEATH INSIDE

If a patient like the one discussed above were brought to the hospital to die, he would, in effect, have had a lingering trajectory outside, concluding in a rapid (or relatively rapid) death in the hospital. A great many patients encountered on hospital wards (especially medical) are traversing such trajectories; they are the majority of terminal patients. Their deaths are relatively uneventful—sometimes virtually unnoticed except by the staff members most directly involved in their care—and they are soon forgotten. If a patient has never before been to the hospital or on the specific ward, if he is almost comatose, if his family is absent or unobtrusive, and if his mode of dying is not unusually unpleasant, painful, or medically exceptional—then conditions are most favorable for the quiet giving of comfort care while the patient uneventfully slips out of the staff's bustling world.

But, change any of these structural conditions, and even these end-of-the-trajectory dyings begin to become more consequential for everybody concerned, the patient included. Suppose, for instance, that an elderly patient is alert, quite aware of what is happening to her, and willing to bow gracefully before the inevitable end of her life; her family also seems reconciled, albeit sad. But suppose also that she is so charming that during her last days the staff becomes quite attached to her. In such an instance, we have seen staff members congregate around a cheerful bedside, laughing and joking, with even the young residents dropping in to talk with "grandma."

Now imagine another elderly woman brought in, virtually dead, "off the street." She is given intravenous treatments and comfort care; but, regaining consciousness and becoming aware of her condition, she begs to be allowed to die. The staff does not fulfill her request. Then she repeatedly removes the IV tubes from her arms, while the nurses just as firmly replace them, until finally, during a period of great activity on the ward, she manages successfully to shorten her life. In this instance (an actual one) the nursing staff was both relieved by her death ("Why should she live, really?") and distressed (though not terribly so) by their inability to prevent her suicide.

If all or many of the structural conditions that contribute to quiet last days are absent, then even a relatively brief period of dying can create great havoc within the hospital. For example, a patient who had been hospitalized several times over a period of six months for diagnosis and treatment reentered the same medical ward for what the staff recognized as his last few days. He had originally been told that he had diabetes, and nobody had ever suggested that he was actually dying rapidly from cancer; indeed, his doctor withheld this information from even his wife until about two weeks before death, suspecting that she could not withhold it from her husband. He proved to be a difficult patient for the staff. To begin with, he was a brilliant young man, obviously destined, if he had not had cancer, for an outstanding career. His wife was overcome with grief, and the nurses were sympathetic. His friends drifted back and forth from the waiting room, with composed but mournful faces—they had finally guessed or been told his fatal diagnosis. These last days were exceedingly painful, and during the last two he became extraordinarily demanding, even insisting on knowing what drugs he was being given, and giving the nurses a generally rough time. He gave no direct sign of knowing that he was dying, but his behavior suggested that he knew but could not accept what he knew.

This complex combination of a difficult but highly valued patient, a tense mutual pretense awareness interaction, the staff's sympathy for his wife, and his physically painful mode of dying made this a distressingly memorable week for the staff. His descent into a final coma, and then death, preceded by brief "snowing" with drugs, could not have come too soon. It left in its wake an exhausted wife and friends, and a disturbed staff.

LINGERING BEYOND EXPECTABLE LIMITS

Whether the deaths involved are easy or difficult, the fore-going instances represent end-of-the-road phases of dying. When the patient arrives on the ward, the staff judges, from well-known physical signs, that he will die rather quickly. The patient him-self, and certainly his family, can also have this expectation. Some-times the physician and the nurses are able to make specific pre-dictions; sometimes they are less certain about the amount of time remaining to the patient, but are prepared not to be sur-prised if he lives a little longer or dies a little sooner than ex-pected. These patients die "on time"—that is, within *expectable limits.*

Some patients who are judged as being very close to death greatly surprise the staff, however, by living beyond their expect-able limits. Their lingering can be very long indeed. At one hos-pital, a patient lingered so long that his insurance ran out. His physician persuaded another hospital to take him as a charity patient, assuring them that the patient would die in just a few days. Then he lingered for months, to the growing dismay of the administrator whose hospital was footing the bill. Such long linger-ing need not greatly disturb the staff, however, if the kinds of conditions discussed earlier are met. A comatose patient does not usually put much strain on the nursing personnel. Yet if such a patient takes too long to die, he may be sent elsewhere while he lingers—usually to a nursing home, but possibly to his own home—because of the effort and expense needed to care for him at the hospital. Or he may be sent to a city or county hospital in order to relieve the family of the expense of his care.

Even if lingering beyond expectable limits is rather brief, it can be exceedingly wearing, even terrible, for family or staff. Oc-casionally, for example, a patient is brought into an intensive care unit shortly after last-ditch surgery, though given little chance for lasting beyond a few hours. If he lingers for even two or three days, his closest kin must wait around until he dies; must readjust their lives to that contingency, making repeated though possibly silent farewells each time they visit his bedside, marking time, so to speak, in their grieving until he has actually "gone." An alert patient in an ICU, well aware of his expectable but briefly delayed death, may plead with nurses to "get it over with quickly"— a request that is not conducive to staff tranquillity.

Another important condition—acceptance of dying—is involved in the following case: A patient had lingered a few days, but her husband did not at all accept her dying. Each successive time that he visited, the nurses found him more difficult to control. They made efforts to cut short his visits to the ICU, and near the end were virtually forbidding him entrance to the ward. When his wife finally died, the husband threw a tantrum in the ICU, throwing himself on the floor and causing unprecedented commotion. More rapid dying would have brought a quite different train of events. Yet a short-lingering death need not greatly upset staff or family, provided the necessary conditions for relative composure are present: no pain, low social loss, or the acceptance of the death by patient and family.

A special case of slow dying within expectable limits arises with the patient who, when first in the hospital, may not be recognized as dying. He has come for diagnosis or simply because he has a known disease that is not expected to be fatal. At some point, however, the staff realizes that "this is it" for this patient: he has only a very short time to live. (This situation is less frequent than another we shall discuss later, when discovery of a fatal illness brings expectations of a much longer time to live— months or even years.) Diagnostic surgery often results in such a sudden revelation. The announcement of imminent death is usually distressing, of course, to family members. They have almost no time to prepare for the loss of their kinsman. The nursing staff is likely to have to cope with family problems, and the physician has to decide whether to tell his patient about his fatal condition. The nursing personnel have an additional problem: they may have become quite attached to the patient, and now he is due to die relatively quickly. The personal careers of some personnel may have become entwined with the patient's, and they have no chance to disengage themselves gradually. In effect, this type of end-of-the-trajectory is a form of slow dying, but it seems to occur quickly after an initial definition that "he is dying." Consideration of this type of trajectory, however, more properly belongs in the next chapter on swift death.

SLOW DYING IN THE HOSPITAL

Among the most complex types of dying trajectories within the hospital are those that are quite properly thought of as "slow" —whether the time of death is certain or uncertain, and whether the patient dies sooner or earlier than expected. Merely to mention those four contingencies, without even bringing in others, such as the degree of social loss, is immediately to suggest the multiplicity of slow trajectories. In the next pages, our efforts will be directed not so much at covering exhaustively all possible types as at focusing on the evolving character of a few but important slow trajectories.

Unpredictability and the Evolving Story

One main property of any lingering trajectory is its potential unpredictability, with regard to both the biological and the human or psychological aspects of dying. To be sure, many a patient slowly declines, or lingers on plateaus between several declines or abrupt deteriorations, without unexpected important events occurring. But in a dying trajectory of considerable duration, a number of special events are probable. Any one can begin to make a special story of the dying. Despite the death, the story may have happy endings for its main characters. Or it may be a very sad story indeed.

The following story was deemed of such human interest that, accompanied by a picture, it appeared in the *San Francisco Chronicle,*[1] six thousand miles from where it occurred.

> Lesly, a physical training teacher [from England], met Jergen three years ago while on a holiday in Copenhagen. A year ago they fixed their wedding day. Soon after, Lesly learned she had leukemia and could never recover. Doctors gave her a final transfusion Friday.

Lesly, however, got married on Saturday, and afterwards had a reception complete with eighty guests, although she "was too weak to cut the wedding cake. . . . Sixteen hours after the wedding the bride was dead. Both knew it would happen that way." Her father said, "It was happiness at the thought of the wedding that kept her alive. Her new husband was at her side when she died."

The reader can only guess at the wealth of detail that went into that story, as day by day the drama unfolded, culminating with her death so soon after the wedding. It seems safe to assume that the couple's decision to go through with their wedding plans was not reached without surprise to the doctors or questioning from their parents. (Later we shall note how a young American who had cancer was advised by his physician not to get engaged in light of "his condition.")

A second instance of unpredictable biological or psychological events evolving during a slow trajectory is recounted in Lael Wertenbaker's moving account of her husband's death from cancer.[2] His malignancy had been diagnosed by a physician in France, where they were living. Tests undertaken in New York City revealed that his cancer was fatal, and he decided to return to France to die. His American physicians attempted to dissuade him, to no avail. His dying ran fairly true to what he had been led to expect, and he managed to keep his increasing pain under good control for some months. There were some unexpected occurrences, but the most unforeseen and difficult contingency was

1. April 13, 1966, p. 6.
2. *Death of a Man* (New York: Random House, 1957).

that Wertenbaker lived some weeks beyond anyone's expectations. Mrs. Wertenbaker's testimonial to his courage arouses sympathy; he drove himself daily to carry on as normally as possible, despite his increasing difficulties in moving about and in maintaining his composure. His story culminates with an attempt to cut short the last days. His first attempt at suicide failed; the second, in which he was aided by his wife, succeeded. In her account, Mrs. Wertenbaker placed her emphasis on a man's living his life until the end as he wished, rather than as a hospital staff might have wished.

In short, both Wertenbaker and the English girl, Lesly, managed to shape their trajectories with reasonable success and personal satisfaction. Wertenbaker's story had a difficult ending, but many unexpected moments of delight. And with very little imagination, one can see that Lesly's story also might not have ended quite so happily.

The slow decline, then, is fraught with both hazard and opportunity. On the hazard side: the dying may take too long, the bodily deterioration may be unexpectedly painful or unpleasant, the patient may discover he is dying when he is not supposed to know, and then "all hell may break loose," and so on. On the other hand, slow decline may allow a man time to make his will, round off unfinished business and family affairs, and even permit somewhat estranged couples or other kinsmen to settle differences. Slow dying also permits staff members to participate in courageous or tranquil trajectories, a kind of participation that buoys them up. All these consequences are less likely to occur with swift or sudden dying.

THE ANALYSIS OF EVOLVING STORIES

Slow dying, then, whether stormy or tranquil, is likely to be accompanied by an evolving story, stretching over weeks or months. The variety of potential stories is infinite, but analytically they can be to some extent reduced to combinations of the variables introduced in this book.

Let us, for instance, look at a rather special "social loss" story, which involves aspects of the biographies of the staff, a patient, and her husband. The patient had been housed at first on a medical ward while her illness was diagnosed. After some weeks, it became certain that she was suffering from a brain tumor. Transfer to a neurosurgical service was followed by an unsuccessful operation. She gradually lost the ability to recognize people or to respond much to them, although she did not become fully comatose for several weeks. The nurses said, "We just kept hoping against hope that she would get better and go home." Nevertheless, "we could see her getting more and more moribund." As she had been a charming, pretty, and talented woman, her gradual decline evoked considerable sadness and empathy for her devoted husband, three young children, and grief-stricken family.

Ordinarily, after such patients "lose their minds," the staff regards them as socially dead, although physically alive, and gives responsible nursing care, but does not take much interest in them. But this woman's story included an unusual contingency. Her husband refused to "give up." He persisted in acting as though his wife might recover. Unlike many other husbands, he visited faithfully every morning and evening until she died; he brought her flowers, read to her, talked to her. "We accepted the fact that nothing we did would help her anyhow, and our personal emotional involvement would have been exhausted at this point, but her husband . . . was so hopeful that for his sake we *had* to, for his sake we *wanted* to give our nursing care towards the end; everything we did for her we were doing for him." And so they succeeded in "prolonging her a little bit, which we felt was undesirable from her point of view but for him it had to be done." The nursing personnel became so involved in his personal drama ("He was one man in a million") that they participated in unusual ways, such as carefully preparing his wife's hair and makeup before his arrival each morning. They also carefully maintained the pretense that she might somehow recover, and guarded against having their composure break down in his presence: "As long as he doesn't break down, you can't; that's the moral obligation you have to him. . . . we couldn't break down as long as *he* kept going."

It is easy to imagine the buzz of conversation among the personnel as they prepared for and later discussed his daily visits and their own actions during those visits. Once they helped him make a decision about whether to let his young son visit the dying mother; they decided "it would do a lot for her and there couldn't be that much harm for the son." One nurse got drawn into this collective ritual of participation and support perhaps even more strongly than the others because she had known the wife and husband back on the medical ward, before the woman was suspected of having a fatal malignancy. But the special efforts of all the personnel, plus the consequences to them, evolved only gradually—in tandem with the development of this complex social-loss story—and could scarcely have been predictable. A final element in the loss story, one that buoyed up the nurses additionally, was their conviction that through their efforts the husband afterwards would never feel as though "something more could have been done." They had done their best, almost beyond the call of duty. And the prolonging of this otherwise "senseless" existence assumed an unusual "sense" through their collective devotion.

The next case was sadder, more devastating by far to the staff, and it illustrates other variables in a slow decline. A teenager, who over a period of years had repeatedly returned to a cancer service, returned once more. One look clearly told the staff that this visit would be his last. Previously a lively boy who teased them and "fought back" playfully, during the next days, Johnnie seemed a completely "changed personality." Patterns of response previously built up toward him were useless. Personnel were perplexed, frustrated, and worried.

> "This time when he came back, he was a changed person," one nurse explained. (She makes facial gestures to show how deeply this hurts her.) When he returned, she was ready for his usual behavior, and asked "Shall I give you your bath?" He said, "Yes, do." She was absolutely taken

aback. The same thing happened when she wanted to bring his food. The next morning, the aide reported exactly the same kind of behavior, and she too was puzzled and disturbed by it. The boy had said he wanted the nurses to know he appreciated what they were doing for him—he had never done this before.

Shortly thereafter he indicated he didn't want to be put in a chair, but wished to remain in his bed.

Two nurses remarked to me [noted the field worker] that with a patient like this, it's so "sad" that you stay away from his room. It hurts to go in and see the change: he is quite literally not the same person any more.

The staff was not able to blame his changed personality on his drug, and so provide a sustaining, explanatory rationale. Shortly thereafter, on the parents' urging, the physician advised the boy against getting engaged to his high school girl because of the chemical treatment he was receiving, as it might have some effect on their children; this advice gave no cues to the boy about his fatal prognosis but, to say the least, did not greatly help his mood.

Two weeks later, the boy had gone through a phase of fighting back, and the staff brightened up at the thought he might be "going back" to how he had acted before; but then he became listless and apathetic again. He also showed signs of growing fear—such as a quivering chin—for which drugs were given him "so we don't talk about it." Increasingly it became evident that "he's given up. He doesn't care what we do, as long as we just leave him alone." In consequence, because he had made quite clear through such gestures that they could do little or nothing for him, the nursing personnel increasingly withdrew from him. They still gave him comfort care, but in relative silence, with few encouraging gestures, and more and more refrained from bouncing into his room to see or speak with him. They could take little pleasure in their care of him: he had slammed a psychological door on them. In effect, he had announced by his actions their uselessness in this period of pre-death. It was not even that he had signaled his preparation for death, so "please respect my privacy;" he had said, "I am essentially dead, so go away."

Two weeks later, the boy's condition had deteriorated so much that his mother began to sleep in his room overnight. His older brother visited and was shocked at Johnnie's changed appearance, thereby upsetting the mother very much. A night nurse comforted her, "Well, you just can't think of everything; it's not really your fault." As the nurse said to the field worker, "You find yourself taking care of the family more than the patient, a lot of times." She had spent several long periods listening to Johnnie's mother pour out her hopes (maybe cancer research would develop a cure quickly) and her grief. One helpful event was that the mother, who by now knew many other patients, had been present when a neighboring patient died from hemorrhaging shortly before her son's death. Afterwards she exclaimed, "Oh what an awful way to go. . . . I'm glad that Johnnie didn't have to go that way." This same young nurse particularly empathized with the youngster, remarking that he wasn't much younger than she. So she wasn't able to feel "motherly" about him, as a nurse should: "I could minister physically and things like this but as far as talking to him about anything, I just couldn't."

In general, this youth's physical decline followed an expectable path: he went fairly rapidly downhill after his last return to the hospital. Nor was the staff's initial reaction to his dying unusual: they had built up an affection for him during his repeated visits, and were prepared to renew the relationship during his final chapter in his story. What was unexpected was his seeming rejection of the staff and their efforts; nurses and aides, and the house physicians, too, reacted with considerable withdrawal. Had the boy accepted his death in a more acceptable manner, with equanimity or cheerfulness, staff reaction would have been very different. Had he talked about his death, or had they drawn him out about his thoughts of death, the course of events would doubtless have been different. Neither party took these steps; instead "mutual pretense" characterized their behavior.

This kind of trajectory is very hard on the staff. Although the death is completely expected and the patient does not die with undue pain, he is so much part of their own biographies and has such great social value ("He is so nice, and so young") that when he makes it plain he no longer wishes their intimacy or their services, they are, as they freely say, "hurt." It is a personal impact, and the wound does not quickly heal. Work obviously suffers, too, if not in quality at least in the quantity of care. A patient like Johnnie is very much what we might term "the patient of the month"—the one who is most talked about. And although other patients may occasionally take precedence in the thoughts of the staff, unquestionably he is a constant threat to the ward's sentimental order. It is almost a relief, albeit a very mixed one, when he dies, both for individuals and for the personnel as a working group.

The trajectories analyzed above indicate how slow dying can give rise to unanticipated dramas.[3] If dramatic enough, these patients' stories are long remembered by people who participated in them. Patients whose trajectories consist of rather unremarkable and expectable events are not likely to have stories spun about their dying. But even trajectories that are fairly uneventful right down to the last phases can produce very memorable stories, as once happened with an elderly lady who was dying slowly according to expectation. Her dying resulted in an especially poignant closing scene because, an alert, aware, educated woman, she was terribly frustrated in communicating her last thoughts and desires. So, too, were people around her as they tried desperately to guess the meanings of her gestures. The story about her dying consisted almost wholly of that closing scene in her life. Yet, in all cases, variable as unexpected events can be, the resulting story may

3. In a forthcoming volume, we intend to present a lengthy case study, complete with analytic commentaries, about a woman who died slowly from cancer. Her increasingly great and seemingly uncontrollable pain was a main theme in her evolving story. Considerable conflict ensued between her and the staff, and among staff members themselves, over the management of her trajectory. The range of consequences for everyone, including personnel seemingly far removed from the ward, astonished even seasoned observers.

always be read as a patterned embodiment of combinations of the key variables (such as social loss, mutual careers, and awareness context) discussed throughout this book.

An interesting feature of the continuing story is that people who have never seen or been involved in the care of a patient sometimes react to his story. In the hospital, some patients generate such memorable stories that they become "personages" not only for personnel who care for them, but also for those who work elsewhere in the hospital. One patient, for example, a nurse dying from a badly executed abortion, roused such feelings in the nursing personnel (most of whom did not know her and had never seen her) that she surely was this hospital's "patient of the month." Another woman set such difficult problems, involving the management of her pain, for the nursing and medical staff that she provoked persistent discussion, which during peak periods of crisis spilled far beyond the confines of the ward: personnel were discussing her story on other floors, in the hospital's restaurant, and even in the classrooms of the associated school of nursing. In the next chapter, we shall see that even patients brought "dead-on-arrival" to the hospital can produce stories to which the staff reacts.

Although strangers react to a dying patient via her story, the reactions of those in prolonged, direct contact with her are necessarily more complex. They cannot simply react to the story; neither do they react merely to the person lying in the bed. It might be said that they react to *a person who is invested with a story.* When the patient groans, requests something, complains, or grows angry at them, their answering actions are not toward isolated behaviors but toward elements of a continuing story. (For example, one difficult patient had a notebook in which she kept meticulous notes about the times when the staff gave her pain medications. The nursing staff increasingly expressed annoyance and anger toward that notebook and when it was lost, they frankly exulted.) A reverse logic implies that a patient's reactions to staff members can be directed toward altering or sustaining the story which they have constructed about him; indeed, a patient may, from his first days at the hospital, deliberately attempt to shape the staff's collective story.

We have seen, then, that patients who die quickly can nevertheless produce dying stories, but patients with slow trajectories are much more likely to have stories that are consequential for their nursing and medical care. As our illustrations have shown, one important consequence of any patient's story—one we dare not overlook—is its influence on the efforts made in his behalf, and thereby (whether we wish to admit this or not) on whether his life will be shortened or prolonged and to what purpose. Stories produced by slow dying are also more likely to have deeper impact on the nursing and medical staffs than those of quicker trajectories.

VI

The Expected Quick Trajectory

The modern American hospital is, above all, set up to handle quick dying trajectories. On the ICU, emergency ward, and operating rooms, medical technology and highly trained staff are concentrated, on constant call, and in a state of constant readiness to meet the challenge of saving—"heroically"—a patient who is dying quickly. "Quick" dying as variously defined by staff may mean within minutes, hours, or a few days.

There are three general types of quick dying trajectories for which the hospital offers several kinds of career. In the *expected quick death,* it is clear to the staff that the patient will almost certainly die in a few hours or, at most, a day or two. The case of *unexpected quick dying, but expected to die* differs in that the staff are certain that the patient is dying, but do not anticipate the early "turn for the worst" and the quick dying that do occur. In a case of *unexpected quick dying, not expected to die,* a patient who has been expected to recover suddenly starts to die quickly, completely surprising staff, family, and other persons involved.

The patient's presence in the hospital provides, from the staff's viewpoint, the temporal basis for defining quick dying trajectories. For example, a heart arrest or the suicide of a "healthy" patient in the hospital initiates an *unexpected* quick dying trajectory; but if these events occur outside the hospital, and the patient is then rushed there, the staff starts off with an initial definition of an *expected* quick dying trajectory. We shall show in this chapter that the impact on the staff of these two cases of quick dying is quite different, even though the end definition—an expectation of rapid dying—is the same. The unexpected quick dying is, of course, much more disturbing, since the temporal basis of medical work and ward sentiment toward the patient is changed abruptly and drastically.

The ICU, emergency ward, premature baby ward, operating rooms, and recovery rooms offer several careers for any quick trajectories, depending on the patient's condition on entry to the hospital, the expected time remaining in the trajectory, and the staff's resources for rapidly redefining the stages of the trajectory in order to help them reverse it or slow it down.

Of five careers we shall discuss, the first three are based on trying to save the patient: (1) The staff may, upon their initial definitions, try to save the patient but after a time redefine his trajectory as the "nothing-more-to-do" stage, and simply *care* for him until death.[1] (2) The staff may work on the patient feverishly, heroically trying to save him until death intervenes, never redefining the initial chance-of-recovery trajectory. (3) Personnel can define the patient as possibly having a quick dying trajectory but also possibly saveable, and then save him; in the end, his trajectory is redefined to that of a recovering patient.

Two careers are based on giving the patient no chance to live: (4) The staff may initially define the patient as having no chance to live or being in the nothing-more-to-do stage of dying, and simply provide comfort care until death, with no effort to save or prolong his life. (5) The staff may have no chance and no time to do anything—even split-second care for saving or for comforting—when they discover that the patient will be moribund in a few minutes or find that he is "going fast."

In this chapter we shall discuss the expected quick trajectory in relation to the structural conditions and social interaction consequences and problems that arise as staff manages these trajectories along one or another hospital career. In the next chapter we shall turn to the unexpected quick trajectory.

---

1. Glaser and Strauss, *Awareness of Dying, op. cit.,* Chapters 11 and 12.

TEMPORAL DETERMINANCY OF SHAPE

Since the quick trajectory is of relatively brief duration, its shape is often quite determinate in regard to time. The staff has a good idea of how long it may take the patient to die, what the ups and downs will be, and what must be done for the patient as the trajectory proceeds. This temporal determinancy of the expected quick trajectory allows the staff to schedule work. In contrast with the atmosphere of timelessness on wards where patients linger, time assumes a solid tangibility on those wards where patients die quickly.

The ability to schedule work becomes a significant factor in the staff's efforts at reshaping (hence redefining) the patient's trajectory while trying to stave off imminent death. They may prolong his life, cause him to linger on, or put him on the road to recovery. This reshaping focuses on the medical aspects of his dying. All manner of equipment, supplies, and staff are kept available on ICU's, emergency wards, and "preemie" wards, for rescuing the patient from death's door or simply managing his physical dying. But reshaping the quick trajectory typically does not affect the patient's style of "living while dying," as it does in lingering dying, when it is so important. For example, the reshaping seldom recoups enough time for experiencing the last days and weeks of longer-term dying, during which so many social happenings occur for patient, family, and staff. It is during these last days and weeks that the patient and his family both prepare themselves for the death; the family makes many visits, takes farewells, engages in last looks; and the staff give comfort care and evolve a story explaining to themselves the patient's impending death, so that it is not so upsetting.

There are several types of expected quick trajectories with fairly clear temporal determinancy. One we may call the "pointed" trajectory. It arises at some point in time when the patient must undergo a procedure that may result in his death—for example, a complex or high-risk operation. The "pointed" trajectory allows the staff to mobilize itself in advance, and to assemble equipment and review procedures that may be required to save the patient. If he is aware of it, the patient with this trajectory is able to bid his family farewell, to sign his own post-mortem certificate, and to say such things to staff as, "If I don't live, this is goodbye," as did one research patient.

Another type is the "danger-period" quick trajectory. In this situation, there is a fairly determinant time period of watching and waiting to see if a patient will make it. If he does not, quick death is likely, although there may be time to try to save the patient or prolong the dying. The staff monitors the patient's condition constantly until the danger is over; for instance, cases of surgical patients in recovery rooms or on the ICU. A nurse said about this, "I think a fairly general statement that is fairly true is that a cardiac patient, if he lives through the first 24 hours, will make it—that's the time when you lose most of them." In some cases, the danger of relapse or reversal may come later, for example, about four days after an organ transplant or brain surgery. Prior to these delayed danger periods, there is often a respite during which staff and family can relax. During the danger periods themselves, everyone involved—staff and family—is totally immersed in the dying situation. The family is in the lounge or corridor waiting for news; the doctor may sit at the bedside for hours watching and waiting. In the case of premature babies, as we have mentioned, the danger period is the first 48 to 72 hours. The nurses carefully watch to see if the baby turns "bad," and a doctor is within immediate contact.

Closely related to the danger-period type of quick trajectory is the "crisis" trajectory. In this case, a crisis that may result in quick death is expected, but it has no defined time of onset or duration. The staff waits. When the prospect of crisis becomes apparent, the patient must be watched continually until his condition changes—either the crisis arrives, or its possibility becomes minimal and can be defined out of his trajectory. For example, if a patient on a medical ward shows signs of going into an adrenal crisis, he is immediately sent to the ICU, to be rescued if the condition develops or to wait until the possibility passes. Some patients come out of surgery with a potential heart attack and are in the crisis trajectory for some days: "It just could happen anytime, so you're prepared for immediate death." In another case, a man came out of surgery for a chest tumor with respiration difficulties and was "closely watched for a couple of days" in the ICU. Recovery rooms and the ICU are the places set up for giving the patient with an expected crisis trajectory a career with the best the hospital can provide in staff and equipment.

A less hopeful quick trajectory is the "will probably die" type. The shape of this trajectory is a steady downhill run to death in a few days. The staff gives the patient little chance, and little effort is made to save him. It is a question of waiting for it to be over and providing such comfort care as is necessary and possible. This nothing-more-to-do situation is typically the result of surgery, an accident, or some physical crisis (heart, diabetic, etc.) that occurs at home or on the street, with the patient brought to the emergency, where it is soon evident that he is too far gone to be helped. One interesting hopeless case is the "inept suicide" attempt in which, for example, the patient puts a gun to his head and shoots it, and the bullet enters his brain but does not kill him. There is nothing to do but, in the words of one resident, "just hook them up to the machine and just wait and wait, and they either make it or they don't." If these cases last a day or more, emergency wards sometimes try to send them to the ICU, with the idea of letting "them" work on the patient.

The "swift" expected trajectory, which may follow a crisis or danger period, is different from those two types because it occurs at the end of a lingering death. The typical case is the cancer patient who has lingered for several months or years with an entry–reentry hospital career, and who with his last reentry may be redefined to a possible quick trajectory. At this stage he does not go to a medical or cancer ward, as before, but straight to the ICU for his last few days. The words of one nurse describes such a trajectory for one leukemia patient: "She'll linger on for some months, then die quickly." With this type of trajectory, unlike the others, the preparations of patient, family, and staff are not left out, since there has been time before the redefinition to expected quick death. But typical end-of-trajectory activities can be missed if the swift death occurs unexpectedly (a heart arrest), for when ample time is expected, everyone, including staff, likes to take their time—sometimes too much—and may not yet be ready for the death of the patient.

All these types of trajectory are potentially changeable into a "save-loss" quick trajectory. This trajectory is not as temporally determinant as the others. In the course of trying to save the patient, the staff succeeds enough so that they do not expect a quick death, they feel he has been saved. Then, suddenly, he starts to die quickly—and perhaps they save him again. This up-and-down shaping of his trajectory can go on for days, resulting in indeterminant expectations as to whether he will live or die. A nurse described one such case briefly: "This man who died last year, one day he was better and the next day he was worse; he was better and worse, and they finally took him back to surgery, and they finally threw up their hands and said they can't do anything." Temporally the work involved in these cases is broken down into small moments that shift the work constantly, each moment being fragile and easily broken into the next. One course of action in work is quickly interrupted for another course.

THE FAMILY

The high degree of temporal determinancy typical in expected quick trajectories usually means that there is family in the nearby waiting room or hallway waiting for news. In the beginning, a nurse or doctor may tell them "everything is going to be all right," but "they know it's not and you know it's not." But time moves very fast in quick dying, and family members must have some explanation to prepare them for the worst. As the patient worsens. the family is briefed by the doctor or a resident; they receive a preannouncement of impending death. This preannouncement carries a tacit agreement that the staff will keep the family posted as often as possible on the patient's condition; and so some family members feel no need to ask questions while waiting. Others want to ask questions as the time plods on, but are afraid—especially if they see the patient with a mask over his face and tubes going in and out of his body, while staff scurries hurriedly around him. Others simply ask whenever they see any staff member, for they suspect from the rapid course of events that by now something must have happened. The usual answer, until the patient has died, is, "He is still not out of danger," thus putting to the family member a temporal orientation toward the dying that indicates he still must wait. In waiting, family members go home, or out for coffee or food. Their return becomes an occasion for asking about the patient, for time has elapsed since they were in contact with the dying and something may have happened. "I just came back from dinner and I wanted you to know," indicates to the staff that the family member is back in contact for information and wants to know if he has missed something while away.

The proximity of the family to the dying patient raises the possibility of the staff's having to manage scenes (which we will discuss more fully in Chapter VII), and also, since a quick death is expected, having to manage the family's desire to be present at the death and/or to take a last look at the patient before or after death. In some cases, the last look or witnessing of death is allowed and is no problem to the staff. "The parents did real well" as they watched their child die under a plastic canopy. In other cases, family members faint upon being lead into the ICU, and must be revived and led away. Some are given a corner of privacy in a room or hallway, so that they may cry and gain control of themselves.

The presence of the family at the bedside during death must be carefully handled by staff since a scene or tantrum is very disrupting to the sentimental order of the ward. Moreover there is real danger that a waiting relative might topple over bedside equipment and harm it or the patient. Some staff members mentioned how, in handling family members of a patient with no chance, they feel embarrassed and helpless because there is nothing to say—unless they simply tell the family it's hopeless.

SAVING THE PATIENT

Providing a quick-dying patient with a "saving career" is an effort made by the staff to change the patient's condition and thus to redefine his trajectory before it is too late. As we have just seen, some types of quick-dying trajectories allow some time and determinant stages for intervening in order to turn the tide; others allow little or no time. Several outcomes are possible if the staff succeeds in reversing the trajectory either into long-term dying or toward recovery. We focus here on the interaction among staff members and between staff and family or patient as these outcomes are produced.

The decision to engage in a life-and-death drama can be complex; sometimes it is delayed or avoided. While the staff of an ICU, operating room, recovery room or emergency room may have the equipment, ability, and time to prevent a quick trajectory from ending in death, the question can easily arise as to whether it is worth it or whether the family would want it. In cases of automobile accidents in which a driver has caused the death of others, the staff may feel an animosity toward him that gives them second thoughts about rescuing him. They may feel he "deserves" to die and that if he does it is "his own fault." The story of his accident becomes a history that, much like a medical history, affects the staff's decisions.

The inept suicide case that ends up on an emergency ward can cause consternation among the staff—to save or not to save. As they go through the patient's danger period with him, some staff members feel that the decision about whether to live or die is properly the patient's: "What are you supposed to do? He should be able to die if he wants to." Other nurses feel that no one should be allowed to commit suicide; ergo, he must be saved.

Some feel that the person who attempts suicide is, by definition. unbalanced and irresponsible, and should be sent to the "psych ward." Moreover, if he dies there it is "his own fault." Thus they redefine his trajectory in an effort to put him on another ward where it is acceptable.

In other cases, the weighty question of whether to save the patient turns on the question of whether to do so would simply prolong the patient's life in a state of sometimes unendurable pain or in one of physical incapability that would make life too much to bear for him or his family. Would the patient simply live on in a comatose state? Would he suffer from severe brain damage? Would he be dependent on machines? Would he be a burden that his family could not physically or financially handle the situation either at home or in the hospital? When the family is consulted, it is not unusual for them to tell the staff that to let the patient die would be "best for all concerned." This is often the case with premature babies or infants with birth deformities. and with severe accident victims, patients with degenerative diseases, or patients whose brains have been denied blood for several minutes. Stories are legion of cases that have been saved at all costs, with the only result being to put the patient in a lingering trajectory of sheer misery for all concerned. Thus, behind the accepted notion that medical staff will try to save all patients, if possible, is a continuous debate among staff members on quick-dying wards that seriously questions how to shape the trajectory for the most humane outcome.

Another element in the decision on whether to save a patient from a quick death is his social value.[2] This is clearly illustrated when limited medical facilities—e.g., a kidney machine—must be used for several patients. The decision becomes, perhaps, less socially biased when a panel of both physicians and nonphysicians decide, although social-value factors still play a part. But in the quick-dying trajectories, when it may be only a matter of hours to a crisis, there is not time to gather a panel, and the staff must

2. See Glaser and Strauss, "The Social Loss of Dying Patients," *American Journal of Nursing*, 64 (June, 1964), pp. 119–21.

decide on priorities. In such a case, the patient's social value may play a strong part in the decision. Age, education, social class, race, marital status, parenthood, and occupation, as well as physical condition and temporal shape of the trajectory become involved in who shall be saved now and who shall be saved later or not at all. Patients are, in effect, competing for life on the basis of their social value. Peak rush hours (*e.g.,* payday night) on wards of city and county hospitals serving lower-class neighborhoods provide good evidence on how the staff judge the potential loss of people to society and accordingly establish their priorities for immediate care.

When the quick-dying trajectory poses a medically interesting problem in saving the patient (*e.g.,* badly burned people) the staff doctor, with little hesitation as to outcome, is likely to try to save the patient. He may try, for practice, even when the patient is not expected ultimately to live, but only, with care, to linger in prolonged misery. But he may also try in cases given no chance, as we shall discuss in a moment.

Sometimes the patient has a moment of awareness that, although he is dying quickly, there is still time to save him, and he screams or simply asks for help before becoming unconscious. One patient who suffered a coronary thrombosis told it this way: "As I was sitting down, an excruciating pain stabbed me in the chest. I gasped, 'Take care of the children, Doris . . . I'm dying. Call the doctor' and I sank into darkness." His wife called the doctor who, under this mandate from the patient, made every effort to save him and did. In another case, a public relations man woke up in the middle of a doctors' conference on how to save him from death and said cheerfully, "Come on, boys, get to work." The doctors, taken aback for a moment, provided him with a career on the ICU that temporarily reversed his trajectory. Such a clear demand by a patient leaves little room for staff decision-making or delays, unless there is clearly no chance.

Sometimes this demand for quick saving comes from a patient who thinks he is at the brink of death, although the staff thinks he will linger. In one case like this, the patient screamed for help and medications to prevent her death, but the staff did nothing extraordinary, and even avoided her. Fortunately for the staff, the patient was wrong. They did, however, leave her on the ICU for four days to help her feel that help was near in case she was right. In another case, a patient who expected to die within several hours asked the nurse to call her husband. Not believing the patient's premonition, the duty nurse asked the head nurse what to do. The head nurse advised calling the husband, just in case. The husband came, and the patient died soon after the farewell. These differential definitions of trajectory often leave little time for reassessment; the disagreement is often hard on both staff and patient, especially because fast action is demanded. and the patient may panic when the staff does not provide it.

In most cases, decision factors balance out in favor of the staff trying to save a patient from quick death if there is time and "some chance." The prime reason, superseding all contrary reasons, is, of course, that saving life is part of their mandate as doctors and nurses. Moreover, even if the patient may perhaps best be left to die, it is easier and safer to prolong life somewhat, and then, under less pressure, consider that alternative. Quick dying generates quick efforts to save, and everyone expects it; lingering dying allows staff more time for decision and more subtle, more covert ways of letting a patient die.[3]

Saving the patient from a quick death brings into play the heroics and life-death dramas for which the ICU's, emergency rooms and operating rooms are well known. Most laymen have seen pictures or heard stories of the doctor working feverishly over the patient, with several nurses and a few other doctors in attendance. The temporal aspects of these heroics in reality vary considerably. Some do involve split-second action—heart massage, for example—but some take hours or days of patient watching and tending. Whether a matter of moments or days, these efforts to save the patient may be construed as a "touch and go" period

3. See *Awareness of Dying, op. cit.*

of his trajectory. In some cases the doctors literally "pull the patient from his grave." In other cases, the patient goes into a save-loss trajectory.

It is at this point in the trajectory that the excitement and challenge of saving a patient grips the staff, and they work long and hard. In the words of one nurse:

> So the doctors were doing external . . . and we engaged in emergency nursing for really eight to ten hours. It was just a question of whether he was going to breathe again or what he was going to do the next time. . . . While all this was going on, there was just so much to do, to have ready, to have there to be used, and so many things that you have to do that [you] don't really think [of] during spare time. This is the emergency situation and you sort of face it. You take a deep breath and say, 'I've done it before and I'm going to do it again. Here we go, you know. Be calm.' Okay, you get past that crisis and tomorrow he's still alive, although the next day I think he's a little slower and more to the dead.

In this case, the man finally died. But after an intense bout like this, failure, albeit marked with a weariness at losing, still carries a clear feeling of exoneration: everyone—the doctors and nurses—did his best with the available skills and knowledge. Success, of course, brings exhilaration, the sense of having pitted human resources against nature and having won.

Sometimes the initial definition of a trajectory indicates to the staff an urgent need for "saving" a patient, when, in fact, he does not need saving. They may work feverishly to rescue him from, say, a heart attack or stroke he does not have. If the patient is conscious, the situation usually requires that he be brought into awareness of his imminent death so that he will let them work to save him. However, a disclosure such as "You may not be *with us* in a few minutes, unless you do what we say" is quite likely to panic the patient.

In one such case, a patient was brought into a hospital with severe chest pains, apparently suffering a heart attack. The staff immediately strapped him down to prevent damage from possible convulsions, and the patient begged to be freed. The doctor, attempting to get his cooperation, explained: "I can't let you out of this thing. You may have convulsions in a minute or two. I can't unloosen these." The patient, realizing the implied quick trajectory toward death, said in panic, "Give me a tranquilizer." The doctor, again attempting to mollify him, explained further: "We can't give you anything. That might kill you." Still more confirmation of his dire prospect came to the patient when a heart specialist arrived, examined him, and said: "You're a very sick man, you know. Would you like to call your wife?" The patient's pain and his panic continued for a few days while the staff watched and tested. Nothing happened, so the patient insisted on going home. The doctors tried to dissuade him but could not. The patient said, "Look, there is nothing wrong with me that you know of. I'm going home." Thus, while the doctors could not redefine his initial trajectory and still justify such a strenuous hospital career, the patient did redefine his trajectory to one that relieved his panic and indicated no need for continued hospitalization. On the basis of the doctors' failure to provide evidence of a real emergency, he withdrew his delegation of responsibility to the staff.

The disparity between professional and lay perceptions of the trajectory did not narrow when this patient returned home. His private doctor remained fixated on a dying trajectory, though a less rapid one. "You are," he explained, "a type of guy who does die, only it takes a little while. I had a case die just like you last week—a reversal." (Doctors do not always change their initial definitions easily, though in this case the new doctor lengthened the duration.) A year later, the patient is still alive, living with his own redefinition of his trajectory, but still panicking when he thinks of what the doctors told him.

This is a good example of a patient who must be brought into awareness quickly, so that the staff can work on him quickly, with minimal interference. But this open awareness context had the unfortunate consequence of leaving the patient with the constant expectation, for perhaps the rest of his life, that he could die quickly any time. Although doctors tend to be cautious about what they tell patients about their trajectories, the work and temporal shape of a quick dying trajectory can lead to unfortunate disclosures to the patients without a prudent consideration of the consequences.

Sometimes, in their rush to save a patient brought into emergency obviously dying, but without a known history, doctors try to save him from an illness that he does not have. There is a risk of not saving the patient (or even of hastening his death) with treatment for the wrong condition. But with only a little time, staff must do something. For example, a patient who arrives comatose and in convulsions may be treated as suffering an epileptic seizure or stroke, when actually he may be suffering some sort of drug reaction. (To forestall this potential mishap, some people carry cards designating their illnesses and medications.) But, all in all, the temporal shape of these trajectories makes action based on an educated guess better than no action at all.

NO CHANCE FOR THE PATIENT

Giving the patient in an expected quick-dying trajectory no chance to live not only reflects his physical condition; it may also say a great deal about the hospital and ward he is in. The trajectory may be one they cannot handle adequately; for example, there may be no oxygen tanks on the ward or no kidney machine in the hospital. Also, as we indicated earlier, social factors may affect whether it is "advisable" to define the patient as having a chance. When a patient is not "worth" having a chance, he may in effect be given none. He may be diagnosed *ad mortem,* rather than treated. Or, as in an emergency ward at peak hours or in an army field hospital in a battle area, he may be given a low-priority designation that proves fatal.

When a no-chance patient arrives on an emergency ward and when there is no time to try anything, the staff's usual maneuver is to put him in a room by himself to die. This is usually a room temporarily available, or space otherwise used for other purposes —a treatment room or office. When the patient dies, the room is again free for its usual use. The doctor, however, may be wrong in determining how little time the patient has, and the extension of the trajectory for several hours may unduly tie up the room. Such an "unacceptable trajectory" puts the staff through an ordeal they did not bargain nor plan for. One nurse, somewhat disturbed by such a lingering, described the following case on an emergency ward: "She was almost dead when we got her, so we just put her into the treatment room and sort of kept an eye on her. There was no sense messing up a bed for her since she was going to die any minute. She died eleven hours later, still on the gurney in the treatment room." Even without staff heroics, then, this patient lingered long enough to suggest the possibility that a more eventful hospital career could have reversed her quick dying. This possibility stuck in the minds of many of the staff.

When there is time, yet clearly no chance of saving the patient, the staff watches, waits, and comforts him until death. They time their comforting efforts according to the progression of his down-hill trajectory, all the while usually remaining alert for a cue that would indicate the possibility of redefining the trajectory to "has a chance." Should this critical juncture occur, they stand ready with equipment and skills to try to save the patient. Staff members constantly refer to the frustration and helplessness they feel while they wait, holding their power in abeyance for a change in the patient that would give them a chance to act.

The following description by a nurse shows clearly how, on the basis of a "flicker of life," a no-chance quick trajectory was redefined, setting in action the work of the staff, which then "resurrected" the patient—a complete reversal.

> The severity of this case was such that these were second and third degree burns, and he was pronounced dead on arrival at the hospital. . . . However, to the amazement of the surgeon, they discovered this little flicker of life, so they operated, and when he came out of four hours of surgery they said "He won't live twenty-four hours," and

his wife said, "We don't know this." He did recover
enough so that he had twenty-five surgical procedures on
his face to replace this missing nose.

This case clearly shows how redefining a trajectory initiates hospital processes set up to change the career of a patient. It also
clearly illustrates "last-ditch heroics." In this case, a physical cue
in the patient's changing condition triggered the effort.

On the other hand, simply because a patient has been given
no chance and shows no sign of a change in condition, the staff
does not, ipso facto, do nothing. If there is *time,* the effort may
nevertheless be made to save, or perhaps only to prolong, his life,
even in the face of very little chance of success. It is not unusual
for a patient to go to the operating table, for example, "with
nine out of ten chances he will not make it through the operation."
Even when they see no chance, the staff recognize the margin
of error in this assessment, as well as the possibility of "miracles."
Hence, when there is time, they may create a chance where there
was none, and organize their last-ditch heroics accordingly.

Last-ditch heroics may be encouraged by several factors. One
is that the patient is of such high social value that his loss must
be averted at all costs. Various forms of these cases appear in
hospitals quite frequently. A prominent person is brought in, in
quick trajectory or starts to die quickly in the hospital. If he is
well known locally, the staff will know his social value; or it may
be by the occupational notation on the record. Even if the staff
does not engage in last-ditch heroics, because it is impossible, or
because they found out the social value of the patient too late, the
reports made to the family, to organizations, or to newspapers are
likely to cast all last efforts—even if purely for comfort—in the
light of heroic efforts to save the patient.

One well-publicized and extreme example of last-ditch heroics
was the case of Dr. Lev Landau, an internationally prominent
Soviet physicist. After a car accident, he was rushed to a local
hospital. The initial definition of a quick trajectory would have
indicated, for anyone else, that there was no chance, and virtually

no time. It was a miracle he was alive when he reached the hospital; he had a fractured skull, brain contusions, severe shock, nine broken ribs, a punctured chest, pelvic fracture, rupture of the bladder, paralysis of the left arm, partial paralysis of the right arm and both legs, and failing respiration and circulation. Within hours, a "who's who" of top Soviet doctors and scientists gathered to provide and "invent" a hospital career that would reverse his trajectory for a time, if not save him. International consultants were called in, and differing definitions of his potential trajectory abounded. Landau "died" four times and was resurrected after each crisis. Several years later, he was still alive and expected to return to work.

This extreme case is mirrored on a smaller scale in desperate cases where the patient has high social value for the local public or for families (such as young mothers or fathers, or children whose social class indicates a good future). Under the pressure of such potential losses, the staff takes every outside chance it can to reverse the trajectory. For example, a little boy hit by a streetcar was worked on until he died; the doctors explored his condition constantly for a possible treatment to save him.

Another, perhaps slightly paradoxical, reason for engaging in heroics, in spite of the impossibility of stemming and reversing a quick trajectory, is the unavailability of a doctor to pronounce the patient dead or define his trajectory in the nothing-more-to-do stage. Thus ambulance drivers may give oxygen to a body until a doctor at the emergency ward pronounces him officially dead. In one case in a small hospital, friends, firemen, and nurses took turns holding the resuscitator to a heart arrest victim until, following extended unsuccessful efforts to find a doctor, a lab technician pronounced the patient dead. A friend said, "We didn't know if he was alive or dead, but this seemed to be the thing to do," especially since the man's wife was just outside the treatment room, expecting him to be rescued. Nurses, too, may engage in quick, last-ditch measures to save a no-chance patient—*e.g.,* heart massage or defibrillation—until a doctor can be found to tell them to end the treatment. Sometimes even a doctor, intensely involved in the patient, the case, or the challenge of preventing death, may engage in heroics after there is no point in them, medically speaking. The inertia of heroics does not let him falter.

A medically interesting patient also stimulates the staff into last-ditch heroics. For example, a patient who underwent an aortic valve insertion operation was expected to die, because the valves often pop out of place. He was hooked into a machine that would signal when trouble occurred—a machine monitoring the crisis trajectory. Although he gave this patient no chance, the doctor worked on him for two or three hours before he died. In this instance, the doctor's concern for the particular patient was reinforced by a desire to find out why the valves tended to pop out.

It is one thing to try last-ditch heroics on a no-chance patient with machines, drugs, and physical procedures; it is another thing to try last-ditch surgery which the patient is not likely to survive. ("We knew before the patient went into surgery that he stood a 90 per cent chance of dying," one nurse said succinctly.) However, it is sometimes the only appropriate procedure left to try. Often it must be done promptly, with the doctor necessarily shouldering the entire responsibility for the decision. If the patient dies, the reason for the loss is sometimes not clear to family members—whether it was the surgery or the patient's condition that resulted in the "table death." Not uncommonly, the surgeon then has on his hands a family that "just went to pieces," and he must explain what happened, covering himself against potential accusations of negligence.

When there is time in the quick trajectory for the family or the patient to participate in the decision to try last-ditch surgery, the choice often hinges upon the relative likelihood that, if saved, the patient will be able to live a normal life. Neither the family nor the patient typically wishes to reverse a trajectory if they recognize that it will unquestionably result in prolonged ordeal or pain.

"Ordeal" is defined in the context of normal life possibilities for the patient. This context includes cultural as well as personal elements, as we can see in the decision of a Cambodian father whose son was dying of gangrene from a leg fracture. The doctor said he would soon be dead from the gangrene, but he would try amputation of the leg. The Cambodian father refused; amputation would render his son worthless for working, a burden to be supported. In America, a father would say "yes" and then get the boy an artificial leg. In India, a lower caste father would also probably say "yes," knowing his son would have a fine career as a beggar (and the operation would be done at no cost).

By and large. American patients or their families—often optimists in the face of hopeless evidence—take the chance: "The doctor told the patient he had one chance in ten of living. The patient decided that that was for him, and so they operated and he's still living." This operation reversed the trajectory for several years. In another case, a patient, although choosing to take the chance, also signed his own post-mortem request, thinking he would not survive. Stories of cases like these are legion in hospitals, and some clearly bring out the general redefinitions of trajectory as they unfold during a hospital career with last-ditch surgery. For example, the patient starts out as "hopeless" in the eyes of staff and proceeds steadily downhill toward death. Unable to stem the trajectory otherwise, the doctor finally, with the patient's approval. takes him to surgery for a last effort to save him, thus initiating a save-loss trajectory. On the operating table. the patient's condition indicates that he cannot survive the surgery. He is sent back to the ward to regain strength and await a better surgical opportunity. As the downward trajectory continues, the staff return him to surgery, saying they will operate anyway. In some cases, they clearly anticipate death on the table; in others, death later on in the recovery room; in still others, a few more days on the ICU with more or with less comfort.

Anticipating the patient's death on the table (that is, defining a "pointed" quick dying trajectory) is a form of preparation for the staff, so that not only will they not be too upset at the death, but they will also understand why extraordinary procedures are being used.

In one case of anticipated death, the surgeon employed two procedures during a heart operation that, to the staff, would clearly have been inadvisable if the patient were expected to live through the operation. However, the patient did live through the operation. The staff nurses then felt that the exceptional procedures had been unnecessary. With sublime hindsight, they held that a patient who was strong enough to support unusual procedures could not have been, as they had been told, too weak to live through a normal operation. The patient, whose quick trajectory changed to a slow but steady downhill run, continued to die for four days, during which the nurses were quite upset. The sentimental order of the operating room staff was seriously disrupted. For four days the nurses came to work all but consciously hoping that the patient had died; each day they were distressed to find him living on, against all the odds. When death came, their initial reaction was that if the patient's presurgery trajectory had been defined "correctly," the operation would have been done "correctly" and he might have lived.

But his death also allowed the nurses to begin to reestablish the sentimental order of the operating room. Death confirmed the view that the patient really had not had a chance; his strong will to live had not been an adequate substitute for a strong heart. The nurses again came to believe that, although his trajectory was not pointed, it was, at least, quick; he had had no chance.

This case also shows how unexpected sudden changes from a quick trajectory to a longer term may be as stressful to staff as the reverse change—because so much action and sentimental preparation is based on the current trajectory, giving staff a stake in the course of action as defined.

THE RESEARCH PATIENT

As we have indicated, last-ditch heroics may employ relatively unusual procedures. In some cases, the quick, no-chance trajectory suggests the use of experimental procedures. The doctor may decide to engage in a research attempt to reverse the trajectory. One approach is simply to try a little-used procedure to see if it will help in this case. Another approach is to put the patient on a research project that needs persons in his condition for developing new procedures (*e.g.*, transplants).

The first type of effort is the epitome of heroics—the last ditch chance that, if it works, is seen as a miracle. A "genius doctor" comes along, gets an idea during the few hours remaining before "certain death," tries it, and succeeds. It is not unusual for these successes to receive nationwide acclaim and full news coverage. Both doctor and patient are pioneers. For example, in one hospital a patient had an unusual, and desperately dangerous, form of heart attack; the heart acquired a bizarre, rapid rhythm. Conventional drug procedures did not work and were reaching the lethal level. One doctor on the case had read about pioneering work on using electric shock to slow down rapid heart beating, though not on such a case as his. He consulted with the patient and family to see if they would agree to try this procedure. They agreed. An enormous electric shock returned the heart to a normal beat, and the patient lived.

Conventional clinical research requires as subjects people who will submit, often as a last resort, to new procedures. Whether successful or not in a given case, the research cumulatively increases medical knowledge and helps mankind. "The patient died, but the operation was a success," if it raises the probability of the next attempt being successful. In one classic case of this sort, the patient gained lasting fame—Marcel De Rudder, the first patient to have an artificial heart implanted in his chest. For him and his wife the operation seemed a final hope, though not a very good one. It did alter his trajectory, a remarkable success for the artificial heart; the patient lingered for five days before dying quickly of a complicating condition. It is typical in these cases that patients are suffering from several conditions at once, while the research focuses on only one. Thus, trajectories may be reversed or slowed down, but only for a time; the patient continues to die of complications.

The De Rudder case is a publicized extreme example of what

happens every day to patients on research wards of hospitals throughout the nation. Patients go to these wards as a last resort ("Nobody else can help me; it's this or nothing") in an effort to reverse a quick trajectory. The basis of this final attempt is awareness and acceptance of the consequences. Some write out death announcements and put them in envelopes ready for mailing, so aware and accepting are they of the potential outcome of this last-ditch hospital career. As they leave for the operating room, some say, "If I don't live, this is goodbye." The nurses say to each other such things as "He'll never make it," or "I hope he'll make it," and make farewell gestures to the patients.

The patient's almost hopeless condition is only one element in the risk-success equation in last-ditch research surgery. The surgeon's experience, both general and specific, is another. And a new procedure is, to be sure, a risk in itself. If the procedure does not work after about ten times, it may be dropped. If successful, it is likely to be turned over to another hospital or ward for further development. Then the research surgeon starts on a new procedure. The research team must be accustomed to "failure" that eventually leads to success, or their sentimental order could not support the high death rate. Too much success, which in these cases is an occasion of great joy and celebration, might reduce the sentimental capacity of the operating team to go back to expecting quick death as the normal state of their research—the acceptable trajectory for a research operating team.

The chief threat to the sentimental order of the surgical research team is facing a bereaved family, even though the families are apprised of the high risk. One nurse said, "I have seen him [chief surgeon] go back to his office in tears from surgery, and not see the family, just be unable to even approach them." Sometimes, when things are not going well, one surgeon or an assistant drops out of surgery to warn the family. These preannouncement interruptions are unusual during surgery using established procedures, because the source of death does not lie so "clearly" in the surgeon's innovative skill.

Moreover, if a surgeon's performance repeatedly indicates lack of this kind of skill, nurses become very antipathetic to his being in research. Their disapproval may even prompt a wave of resignations. To be sure, it is acceptable to have patients die quickly on the table; but table deaths are not acceptable for reasons of incompetence. The patient should die from his condition, coupled with a yet unperfected procedure, but not from bungling.

We have chosen to discuss research surgery because its immediate effect can be to reverse the trajectory of a person only hours from death. Drugs can also, in a matter of hours, stem a quick trajectory. but usually they take longer. Clinical research with drugs is more applicable to the lingering "nothing-more-to-do" dying patient, for there is more time to study the drugs' effects.

VII

The Unexpected Quick Trajectory

As noted in the beginning of Chapter VI, two kinds of unexpected quick dying trajectories are relevant to our discussion of the relationship of staff work and the sentimental order to the course of a dying trajectory. One is the unexpected quick trajectory of a patient already perceived as dying; the other that of a patient not previously considered as dying. (Since these trajectories are defined in the hospital, the *unexpected* quick dying of a "healthy" person, as in an accident, is defined as an *expected* quick trajectory upon entry to the hospital.)

Much of what we have said about the expected quick trajectory applies also to the unexpected trajectories, as will be apparent throughout the chapter. The principal difference between the two types is their impact on the work and sentimental orders of staff, who usually are less prepared for the unexpected trajectories. Therefore, we shall focus principally on those "surprise" features, which tend to apply only to the unexpected trajectory.

EMERGENCY OR CRISIS

A crucial structural condition in the hospital staff's handling of an unexpected quick trajectory, whether or not the patient is already considered as dying, is whether the "surprise" comes as an emergency or as a crisis. The two situations typically have different impacts on staff work and sentiment.

An unexpected quick trajectory requires immediate mobilization by the staff for the effort to reverse its drastic end. The *emergency* situation almost always implies that the facilities for mobilization of quick action are at hand and that prompt action can be initiated at a moment's notice. In the *crisis* situation, on the other hand, adequate preparation for mobilizing quick action is often lacking, so that the need to act immediately more or less immobilizes the staff. The work and sentimental orders suffer accordingly. In the emergency situation, the staff recovers quickly from surprise, mobilizes immediately, and promptly achieves a solid feeling about what is happening. In the crisis situation, the relative disarray of work and sentiments requires a much longer period for working itself out before the work and sentimental orders are solidly reestablished.

Whether a situation becomes crisis or emergency depends largely on several initial conditions; others may become pertinent as the situation unfolds. As we have explained earlier, specific hospital wards are prepared to handle particular kinds of trajectories. The unexpected dying trajectory that occurs on a ward that is capable, in terms of facilities and personnel, of coping with it is considered an emergency, and a career to stem the quick dying is immediately mobilized. Although the particular case presents an unexpected trajectory, the ward is geared to this type of trajectory, can predict what will happen, and finds it acceptable. As we have noted, the concentration of staff (especially doctors in attendance) and equipment on the ICU's or emergency wards makes them suitable places for emergencies. Around each bed on an ICU or in a recovery room are the machines necessary to manage the patient's environment in relevant ways at a moment's notice.

On most other wards the unexpected quick trajectory is typically unacceptable because immediately available resources are not adequate to handle it. The appearance of the unexpected quick trajectory constitutes crisis. On these wards there is no general preparation for quick dying trajectories—at least of certain kinds—and the work and sentimental orders of the ward "blow up" when they occur. A career adequate to the situation cannot be mobilized fast enough, and the patient must be whisked to the ICU "before it is too late." The staff on the less-prepared ward is also likely to be faced with handling a seriously disturbed social situation among patients and family members, which is unusual on wards geared to the unexpected dying, where quick mobilization focuses the social situation for all parties. Family members on less-prepared wards must be handled so as to prevent or to cope with their "surprise" and their scenes (crying, even tantrums) in front of others. Other patients must be calmed down, and prevented from seeing what might or could unexpectedly happen to them. The staff must collectively help itself to regain sentimental balance.

An unexpected dying situation or a death on a ward that seldom experiences such a case can leave nurses or doctors in shock for some time (see Chapter II). In one case, it was the the death of a delivering mother. In another, it was heart arrest in a patient who was being worked on for routine reasons. Patients sometimes die, or start to die, during routine operations because of an unanticipated response to the anesthesia or to the operation itself. Before the "natural causes" can be discovered and combated, the surgeons may be subjected to severe accusations of negligence or bungling by other members of the staff. Sometimes the accusations prove correct. In one strange case reported in a newspaper in England, an unexpected quick dying trajectory resulted in the death of an adolescent on the operating table. It was discovered he had been over-anesthetized by a doctor who was an anesthetic addict. He took a whiff himself, dozed out, and inadvertently killed the boy.

But even wards with high mobilization potential have limitations on which unexpected quick dying trajectories are manageable. Thus, in spite of staff professions that "anything can happen in Emergency or ICU," it is clear that not "anything" can be handled readily, and that some unexpected dying trajectories can still cause a crisis situation on these wards. We learned, for example, of one crisis that arose when a patient who unexpectedly started to die on an ICU was quickly hooked up to an oxygen outlet on the wall, but kept right on dying. When he did not respond, the staff went into crisis on what to do for this strange condition. Later, after death, his failure to respond did not prove so strange; the oxygen outlet had been connected to an empty tank.

Even "routine-emergency" procedures can generate crises. When a needed doctor or skilled member of the staff is not in attendance, an emergency situation may shift to a crisis. For example, an ICU patient's heart stopped. It would have been a routine emergency for the surgeon to do open-chest heart massage, but he could not be found, and none of the staff present could perform the task sufficiently well.

Sometimes the ward does not have the necessary equipment for a particular emergency (*e.g.,* a kidney machine for renal failure) although it is prepared for other unexpected quick dying trajectories. Sometimes the mobilized action involves use of a machine that breaks down, and a routine emergency turns into crisis. In one such case, the staff tried to stem the crisis by borrowing a similar machine from another patient, who herself would not need the machine before the breakdown was repaired.

Sometimes the ward has facilities and skilled personnel for handling an unexpected quick dying trajectory on an emergency basis, but cannot mobilize themselves to act in time, and so a crisis occurs. In these cases, the sentimental order is so disrupted by the "surprise" that mobilization stops. One case that paralyzed an emergency staff into crisis was the shooting of the ward clerk by a former lover, a deputy sheriff who was bringing a patient to the ward. Staff members were so shocked that they could not at first begin the routine for standard unexpected emergencies. They gaped and mumbled: "She was one of us." "It's different when it happens to an employee of a hospital." "We knew her and it's harder to lose someone you know." "Sheriffs don't do that." As the nonmedical features of this surprise subsided, and the staff could again see pertinent medical aspects of what had happened, they could start to shift the crisis back to routine emergency treatment of a bullet wound. However, they were too late to save the patient.

Even on a ward geared for emergency, differential definitions of a patient's trajectory by two or more doctors can also forestall mobilization for the best course of action and thus generate crisis. These disparate views of the patient's condition can filter down to the nurses, who are relatively immobilized by such uncertainty about the type of procedure they are told to apply. Their motivation is undermined by the lack of a clear course of action, and their fears that what they are doing for the emergency may precipitate a crisis may be well founded. These cases occur particularly when a patient comes into an ICU or emergency ward with no history, will not or cannot give one, and unexpectedly starts to die. Something must be done quickly. Mobilization itself produces crisis as the staff, not knowing what is actually wrong, and divided on what to do, mobilize in different ways. Very often the answer is not discovered until the post-mortem, or later diagnosis of recovery; sometimes it is never discovered at all.

Other cases of crisis occur on wards where an unexpected quick trajectory is acceptable, but the surprise goes unnoticed until there is either no chance to save the patient or he has died. Mobilization ability is of no avail. We have already mentioned several conditions of the ICU, emergency ward, or preemie ward that allow such unexpected cases to go unnoticed; for example, another urgent case is receiving all the staff's attention. The shifting priorities of care may also disarm the staff. Moreover, a surprise by its very nature may go unnoticed for hours—for instance, if it arises early in the interval between routine checks on the night shift.

The hospital itself can generate conditions that produce an unexpected quick trajectory for which it can provide no emergency career, only crisis. In one such case in a small suburban hospital, a patient on his way to surgery for a routine procedure was killed when an elevator started to go up while the gurney was only half way through the door; there was no safety "stop" button. Or on understaffed wards, patients in isolated sections are able to take their own lives without being observed.

THE IMPACT OF SURPRISE

As we have noted, the unexpected quick trajectory's surprise impact on the staff varies in degree according to whether the patient has previously been considered as dying. Generally the surprise is more complete when the patient has not been so considered. However, the structural conditions surrounding each dying situation can affect the surprise impact considerably; and these conditions set limits on how the staff reinstates its sentimental and work orders.

Some Degree of Surprise

When a patient is expected to die, but not quickly, the staff attempts to anticipate the timing of his trajectory as specifically as possible. They then work and develop sentiments according to the temporal stages of the trajectory. They expect to see the patient for some time to come, and expect warning signs as he moves into each new stage of dying, cues that indicate he should be watched closer, that he should be sent to the ICU for constant care, and so forth. They anticipate the family's becoming more and more prepared, and thereby more cooperative or less bothersome.

On medical wards, when an unexpected quick trajectory begins in a lingering patient, expected stages may be entirely left out of the dying, or may be hurried through as fast as possible. For example, the family, as yet unprepared, must be found and told that their relative is almost dead, an often shattering task for the nurse or doctor as well as for the family. Staff work and sentiments lose their customary tempo and continuity. Mobilized for slower paced dying trajectories, the staff may lapse into momentary crisis because of the unexpected "swift" dying. Sudden procedural shifts may be required. Facilities must be obtained quickly and the right doctor found, or the patient must be moved to the ICU. If the patient remains on the medical ward, extra nursing staff must be found to help with other patients until the crisis can be turned to an emergency; for the medical ward is most likely to be understaffed for such occasions, their quota of nurses being based on routine, slower paced care.

Having become personally involved in the patient and his family, the nurses may suffer some shock at the dying. Over time, some nurses may also have come to expect the lingering patient to be alive each day they arrive on the ward. They expect to greet a familiar face; for the time being they forget he is dying. One patient on a pacemaker lived five years, during which time he repeatedly returned to a medical ward for checkups. Although the nurses knew he could die in a moment, they got so used to seeing him they just expected him to go on living. When he died from a corroded wire, it was a shock to all the nursing staff.

On the other hand, the unexpected quick trajectory may be well received on the medical ward. If a patient has been lingering in pain, has been degenerating, has been comatose for months, is draining his family of all their money, has clearly reached the nothing-more-to-do juncture in his dying trajectory, with nothing to make his last weeks and days socially meaningful or even comfortable, the staff may wish that he be allowed to die. Or they hope, sometimes quite overtly, for a change in his condition that will put him in a quick dying trajectory. They may, in effect if not in conscious intention, allow a failure in the equipment that is prolonging his life to put the patient in a pointed quick trajectory—a tube falls out and is not replaced fast enough, a patient is not suctioned in time. However, it is circumstantially as well as "morally" difficult to engage in overt tactics that initiate a quick dying trajectory. The correct conditions of nonvisibility and permitting circumstances are unusual in hospitals, except perhaps on night shifts. The following statement from a nurse must be taken as indicating that while the sentimental order of medical wards can, under some conditions, condone an unexpected quick trajectory (much as it can intensify the surprise at one), the work order usually cannot sustain the necessary action to initiate it. "When she [the patient] tells me that 'I want to die,' it's at that point that I will go right up and say to the doctors, 'Let her die.' "

Although the presence of dying on medical wards may be common, death itself may be rare. The sentimental order is not geared to death, especially to sudden death from a quick trajectory. At worst, the staff expects to have time to prepare for anticipated death. Not having experienced many deaths, they are not so well protected from the surprise of quick dying as the staff on the quick-dying wards. In many of the dying cases, they expect the patient to meet his death on other wards or in an isolated room on their ward; but with the unexpected quick trajectory, there may not be time for such a move.

On the quick-dying wards, the greater frequency of deaths tends to temper nurses for the surprises as well as for the expected. A surprise can be warded off: "We generally lose them anyway." One ICU nurse clearly indicated how the sentimental order of the ICU is capable of handling all deaths, including unexpected and sudden dying. When asked what kind of a day she had had, she responded, "It wasn't so bad; at least we didn't lose anybody today." This ward had had a death every day for five days in succession.

Generalized protection against the surprise of an unexpected quick trajectory is sustained by other facets of the quick dying wards. The dying patient would have lasted only a few days anyway, so the temporal loss is not great. The unexpected quick dying may be welcome relief from bearing even a few more days of an ordeal painful to all. The quicker death also maintains the ward personnel's motivation to rescue patients, by relieving them of a "no-chance" patient sooner than expected, and opening a bed for a patient who can be saved.

On quick-dying wards such as the ICU and emergency, the intense work and the intense focus on medical aspects of saving also provide buffers to unexpected dying. Staff have no time to dwell on the surprise and the sad fact of imminent death, as they do on the medical wards. Rather they must concentrate on mobilizing for the emergency and preventing crisis. When asked to remember such a case, one nurse had a hard time, for forgetting is easy when the concentration on rescue is so immediate and intense. She said, "I don't question, I really cannot, I haven't got time to think about it while I'm doing things," following this with a description of trying to save the patient. Involvement is more in giving medical care, and not so much, as on the lingering wards, in feeling about the patient. Another nurse explained: "There's always so much involved in trying to save the patient's life, but you don't have time to think about your own feelings, and then it's so terribly realistic that once it's over, then you have this letdown feeling, but nonetheless it's a realistic one, I mean the man is dead and that's it." The death, surprise or not, is accepted, and the nurse goes on to another patient.

Part of this intensity in medical care involvement is induced by the close collaboration of work with the doctor, an ideal seldom achieved by nurses on the medical ward. When an unexpected quick dying trajectory appears on the ICU, emergency, or operating room, doctor and nurses quickly join forces for the emergency. Nurses take on much responsibility in treatments, and derive great satisfaction from their part. In one such case, the doctor, after rescuing a patient from the unexpected, said in the presence of others, "If it hadn't been for the nurses, this man wouldn't be alive." The nurses repaid his praise by commenting that, after all, he had put in "the gadget." The sentimental order of these wards is also bolstered by general statements such as "This kind of work is probably the most important area of nursing."

The intense work of quick-dying wards is generally supported also by adequate staffing and facilities suited to emergency handling of the unexpected. Sufficient doctors and nurses are on hand or promptly accessible. Those engaged elsewhere know how to shift quickly to a patient who suddenly starts to die. For example, one nurse, reporting on a recovery room where patients may unexpectedly start to die from their surgery, explained in a somewhat exaggerated statement: "It's the one place in the hospital where the critically ill have a chance to survive because he's got people who know what to do in an emergency, and he's got equipment and facilities available." Moreover, staff can cope with surprise dying with aplomb because the patient has usually not been on the ward long enough for personal interest to have developed. Also they are well insulated from the family, who might otherwise arouse their concern; the staff work behind closed doors, and the family is kept in a waiting room. These protective circumstances are strongest for operating room teams.

Several aspects of the patients themselves can, however, break through the protection against surprise afforded by the work and sentimental orders of the quick-dying wards. A patient of apparent high social value may penetrate the nurses' immunity to surprises. One ICU nurse said, "I took care of a young boy who was a medical patient and who was comatose when I came on. He expired after my shift. When I got the news that he died suddenly, I felt badly, and I still feel badly and I don't really know the whole story." Nurses have a generalized feeling for the loss such patients create for others, a feeling based on what kinds of people society values most highly.

The unexpected death of the medically interesting case also may disturb nurses. One ICU nurse illustrated this clearly when asked about a patient who had died on the evening shift. She had forgotten who he was, and nobody else remarked about his death. Then she said, "There wouldn't be too much to say unless it is an interesting medical case. When a patient is interesting medically there's a lot of talk about him, and that's one of the reasons why people will get involved or interested in certain patients." The intense involvement in work can in turn generate a personal involvement in the patient in these cases.

Along with a patient's social value or interesting condition, the staff's "investment" in him can ruin the generalized protection afforded staff (particularly nurses) on quick-dying wards. We see this in a comment about the sudden death of a high-risk patient who had little chance: "The doctor has worked so hard to save him." What reaches the nurses is the doctor's loss, not the patient, who "was never a person to me." The object of concern and distress is the doctor. In the words of another nurse, "I'm sorry for the doctor because of the time and the effort, and I'm sorry for us because we spent an awful lot to help this man live." Often the high-risk patient is also medically interesting, which is why he is offered a saving career even though there is little chance: "I'm interested in him because of the type of surgery he had, which is new and different." Thus, the accumulation of a work loss and a concern for a doctor who probably worked hours on the patient increases the impact of surprise on nurses if the patient suddenly dies, even though he had little chance.

This cumulative impact can be compounded further if the patient also suddenly dies for the "wrong" reason. The report of one nurse emphasizes this in the case of a high-risk, high-investment, medically interesting patient: "I was frankly quite shocked when I had come around the corner and the patient had died. Dr. X was there when the patient died, and apparently had been trying to avert it. It turned out that he had not died from having the plug pop. Dr. X said he didn't know what he died from."

Nurses may handle surprises such as these with several ready rationales, so standardized as to comprise a ward armamentarium of defenses for its sentimental order. For example, "There are only so many complications that one can live a life with, and he had too many." Or, "I think, since he did have several complications, it was probably better for him and his family that he did die."

Certain staff members' surprise may be increased by the patient who provides them a rehearsal of dying. Rehearsals occur in most cases of dying, but the sudden quick trajectory can make them more startling. One nurse said, "The patients who concerned me most when they died were women of my own age, and these very often were cardiac patients who went into surgery and didn't return." In this case, the nurse was rehearsing what could happen to someone like herself. Other patients who provide rehearsals are those who have diseases similar to (though further advanced than) those of nurses or their relatives.

INSTITUTIONAL EVASIONS

A nurse under the pressure of an unexpected quick trajectory, may be made momentarily helpless to avert it by several circumstances. The surprise catches her unprepared, but she jumps to mobilize an emergency treatment. There she finds herself unable to effect the mobilization because she is forbidden by law to give the necessary treatment, and the doctor in charge is inaccessible. The situation approaches crisis. At this point, surprise and helplessness can force her, if her actions will not be visible, to evade institutional rules of the hospital or of medicine.

This configuration of conditions occurs on all wards, but is less likely on the quick-dying wards where finding another doctor is easier. Something must be done quickly when sudden dying starts. Sometimes the available doctor is not prepared or not skilled enough for some of the uniquely complex cases one finds, even on the ICU or in the recovery room. As one nurse from the ICU affirmed, "If a resident is called from the nearby medical ward, he may do something wrong, and it is usually the nurse who is blamed for it." In other cases, a doctor capable of saving the patient may be loath to work on another doctor's patient, especially a private case. At this juncture it is not unusual for a nurse to take the situation into her own hands and treat the patient. Many of these evasions of the rules are minor; for instance, an injection into the circulatory system may sometimes be informally ordered by the doctor in case of sudden changes while he is unavailable. The nurse is not held accountable for them if they are discovered.

However, on the quick-dying wards, particularly the ICU, institutional evasions can take on a serious dimension. The complexity of some cases means that only the doctor in charge has the right skill—and the right—to save the patient. To prepare for unexpected changes when he is unavailable, this doctor may train his nurses to treat the patient. In essence, he trains them for institutional evasions that might, if death follows, bring them severe consequences—dismissal, accusations of professional negligence, or a manslaughter charge. The doctor and the head nurse support nurses in these evasions; on the other hand, the nursing supervisor distant to the ward may not endorse such action but can usually find no alternative, except letting certain patients die. Given no alternatives, conditions combine to force nurses to engage in institutional evasions; and nurses tend to act because the work and sentimental order of the ward support any course of action that tries to reverse an unexpected quick trajectory. Nurses may give an adrenalin shot directly into the heart, or engage in open-heart massage. They have something to do to handle their surprise and the pressure on them, and the ward provides an immunity from punishment.

COMPLETE SURPRISE

In general, the greatest surprise impact from an unexpected quick trajectory occurs in the case of a patient who was not expected to die, but who was, indeed, expected to make a complete recovery. The essence of the complete surprise when a recovery patient goes into a quick dying trajectory is the low probability of such a reversal, although, as one nurse said, "Everyone knows that this could happen, but it only happens once in umpteen times. This kind of death is very upsetting to everybody." Her statement referred specifically to the explosion of the anesthetic in a patient's chest, but it could just as well apply to any other source of unexpected quick dying in hospitals—suicide, drug effects, heart arrest, hospital accident, respiration difficulties, etc. As we saw in Chapter II, if the patient has been on several wards, a good portion of hospital staff can become distressed over the sudden death of a patient on the mend.

The impact of complete surprise varies from ward to ward. In spite of the shock, staff on the quick-dying wards are better able to mobilize for such emergencies. On medical wards, where the staff seldom experience such quick, unexpected dying, they may find themselves without either emotional or medical strategies for rescuing the patient—and crisis results. The unexpected quick dying we observed on an obstetrics ward caused pandemonium among staff; it was clearly an unusual, unacceptable trajectory for this ward.

In an unexpected quick-dying trajectory of a recovering patient, the question of staff negligence can easily be raised. The patient or his family has delegated the management of recovery to the hospital staff. To learn that he is dying fast (or is dead) makes them reconsider that intention. It is not hard for them to suspect some kind of negligence and, if death occurs, to start voicing accusations. In the United States, there may be threats of coroner's inquiries and malpractice suits. In Italy, relatives may have tantrums right on the ward, in front of all the patients. In Greece, as we noted earlier, one family stoned the hospital windows.

Indeed, staff members themselves may level accusations of negligence at coworkers, or at themselves. Self-accusation may be revealed indirectly, as with a doctor who lost a patient during a simple operation and was so broken up he could not operate for the rest of the day. Another doctor who lost a mother in the delivery room broke down and cried.

Instances of accusing others sometimes reveal more about the accusers than about the accused. One such instance was the case of a child who had heart surgery and was not supposed to die; but the child got a staph infection and did die. The shock was even greater because of the great social loss. In private the nurses accused the physician of using contaminated equipment, an extremely tenuous, emotional attribution. Sometimes, however, the basis of the accusation is less ambiguous, as when a post-surgical patient almost hemorrhaged to death because the surgeon forgot to tie off an artery before closing the incision. Again staff accusations flew. Presumptions of negligence occur on all wards, but stories involving operating room and ICU personnel perhaps are most frequent. Besides accusing the doctors, nurses sometimes

blame each other, or themselves, for not picking up early symptoms or signs, or for not believing them serious enough to report
to the doctor.

Accusations of negligence toward self and others revolve
around errors—real, suspected, or imagined—of either omission
or commission. Errors actually committed usually seem to the
staff to be more drastic, but errors of omission are no less deeply
felt when sudden quick dying results in death. The suicide made
possible because of the patient's isolation or neglect by the staff
is hard for the staff to accept. They may spend hours debating
what they saw and did not see, how he might have asked for help
in a way they did not hear, what truly was their fault and what
was just unfortunate. (We discuss post-mortem stories about patients at length in Chapter X.) Doctors will ask, even demand,
autopsies of the suddenly dead in order to discover what happened
—that is, how much their competence is at issue.

Seldom do these debates, attributions of error, and accusations
of negligence get beyond the non-visible, behind-the-scene aspects
of medical care; thus seldom is anybody actually held publicly
accountable.[1] Moreover, many of the errors are social-psychological and, therefore, are not officially held accountable even
when visible. But whatever the nature of the error or neglect—
real or imagined, attributed to self or to others—accusations
break up the sentimental order of the ward and may upset the
work order. Doctors grow even more than normally hesitant to
assist in colleagues' cases, or indecisive in their own. Nurses insist, even more than usual, on explicit instructions, hesitate in
supplying the doctor with requested items, or temporarily lose
their composure completely.

Reinstating the Sentimental Order

In reinstating a satisfactory sentimental order to the ward,
the staff employs a number of strategies, several of which we have

1. See Anselm L. Strauss, Barney G. Glaser, and Jeanne Quint, "The
Nonaccountability of Terminal Care," *Hospitals,* Vol. 38 (January, 1964),
pp. 73–87.

already mentioned. In general, these devices involve feeling differently about a dying patient and working differently with him. Salutary changes are often instituted by redefining his trajectory to quick dying and altering his hospital career. The staff then know better what to expect, what to do, and how to feel toward this patient and his family. These new clarities feed back into the disturbed sentimental order of the ward, becoming the new basis of an improved sentimental order more in line with what may happen on their ward, and what they must do when it does happen.

The redefining of the trajectory may be self-evident and spontaneous. Or it may depend on explicit statements and actions of the doctor or the nurses. Once the redefinition starts, it is worked over by talk among the staff. They clarify, explain, and recognize the consequences of the quick trajectory for the patient and for their work and feelings. For example, they may "humanely" conclude that it would be better for him and his family if he were to die quickly. Then they develop a new story in support of their new view, and respond to this story rather than to the patient as the essential ingredient in the sentimental order. This process and its effects are evident when a nurse who never knew the patient but is quite disturbed by his sudden dying on her ward is calmed by being told of the new trajectory and story.

Reinstatement usually starts promptly. During quick trajectories staff members immediately grasp for any possibility to help them regain composure. Little or no negotiation of redefinitions occurs at first. Typically, one key person—the nurse or doctor on the scene—initiates the redefinition, and the rest fall in line. Refinements of the redefinition or accusations of negligence get worked out later, if at all. If the reinstatement proves sustaining for staff, and the story can be laid to rest, nothing may ever be said again. Uncertainty about a drastic change in trajectory or an error is the condition for later discussion; clarity about the change and its explanation brings quick closure to further group talk about the case. And reinstatement of a satisfactory sentimental order provides for the staff a modified and broadened repertoire of responses, rationales, and strategies for future dying situations on their ward. Each temporary breakdown constitutes a preparation for forestalling future breakdowns.

Redefining the patient's trajectory leads to reorganization of work (in this case, mobilizing for an emergency) which, as we have said, feeds back to reinstating a favorable sentimental order. The staff have new expectations and feelings about what can now be achieved for the patient, and get on with doing what they can. But reorganization of work affects the sentimental order in other ways, too. As all become informed of the new trajectory in some manner and degree, new relationships develop among staff members and with the patient and family. New groupings of personnel (*e.g.,* intense doctor-nurse collaboration for saving) emerge for different treatments to the patient. New problems arise in handling family members. They, too, may need treatment (*e.g.,* sedation or comforting talk) or may be given work in caring for the patient, such as watching him closely and constantly. New people may be called in—a specialist for the patient, a chaplain to work with the family or patient. Other patients whose own care may have been delayed or changed during the crisis again receive their routine care. As this reorganization of work takes hold, the sentimental order of the ward stabilizes at a new "normal" level.

SUICIDE IN THE HOSPITAL

Two kinds of unexpected dying trajectories illuminate these themes of handling the shifting work and sentimental orders of a ward with particular clarity: suicide, and death on the operating table.

Suicide in the hospital is almost invariably unexpected. Even if its possibility has been anticipated, steps will then be taken to prevent it, and the staff no longer truly expect it.[2] Staff classify these unexpected suicides or suicide attempts that put a patient

2. There is one exceptional situation, which we have discussed as the "set-up for auto-euthanasia" in our *Awareness of Dying, op. cit.,* Chapter 12.

into a quick dying trajectory in two ways, according to their importance to themselves: could or could not have been anticipated. The suicide that can be anticipated is usually "reasonable"—*e.g.,* the patient was riddled with cancer. Its reasonableness leads the staff to feel that there were justifiable grounds for taking one's own life. It is hard not to accept as reasonable justification a suicide note such as this: "Since Thursday I have been in such extreme pain that no amount of medication will bring it under control." In view of the presence of conditions "justifying" the suicide, it *could* have been anticipated by staff members.

The impossible-to-anticipate suicide comes completely out of the blue. There seems no forewarning reasonable justification for such extreme action. Later review of the patient's story may render the act understandable (see case in Chapter II); but this understanding does not constitute a reasonable justification that, in the staff view, could have forecasted the attempt. For example, a psychological condition such as loneliness at night, which might lead to suicide, may make the suicide understandable afterwards, but it is seldom an occasion for preventive measures, except perhaps in a psychiatric hospital or by nurses with a strong psychiatric orientation. To most staff members, "reasonableness" depends on severe physical conditions that appear intolerable.

Even with physical condition as the criterion, anticipation depends on the nurses, who vary in their ability to recognize a potential suicide. For example, one night nurse twice prevented a man from committing suicide. After her shift, she told the head day nurse to watch for further attempts. The head nurse replied: "You're an alarmist. He certainly doesn't want to jump out of the window. There's no reason for you to say such a strange thing. Go home and go to sleep." The patient, unattended, jumped out of the window a few hours later!

After a suicide trajectory (whether or not death is the outcome), differences in anticipation are battled out in the postmortem story that develops about the patient's case. Staff members thoroughly discuss the physical, psychological, and social indications on which they were basing their anticipations. "The patient put on a nice front." "The patient didn't seem to be in much pain." The staff then ends up with a balance sheet of cues in favor of whether a suicide attempt should or should not have been anticipated. They also may have learned much about what to watch for in future cases.

To anticipate a suicide attempt is to define a potential dying trajectory, setting in motion preventive measures that alter the patient's hospital career. He may be sedated or tranquilized. Drugs are put out of reach. The doctors may initiate a search for any weapon the patient may use on himself. The nurses go through the patient's belongings for weapons, "feeling very phony." If a weapon is found, the doctor may confront the patient with it, letting him know the staff is on to his plan, and trying to talk him out of it. Or staff may threaten to send him to the "psych" ward. They may institute a constant watch, which means a loss of privacy for the patient; e.g., they pull the screens back from around his bed so that all nurses can watch as they move around the ward.

A strategic part of the potential suicide's new career is being taken out of any "suicide space" and kept from slipping into one unnoticed. "Suicide space" is any place in the hospital that "allows" or "encourages" the act. It provides an area of nonvisibility. It provides weapons, such as razors in a bathroom. It provides means, such as bathtubs in bathrooms, or drugs on pharmacy carts, or unbarred windows in unobserved parts of hallways. If the patient is in or has easy access to a suicide space, he is transferred to a ward where the possibility of reaching a suicide space is minimized and he can be easily watched. If he must go to a suicide space—to the toilet, or downstairs in an elevator—an orderly or aide is sent with him. If the patient suddenly cannot be unaccounted for, the staff search for him immediately. In one case, a nurse looked up, glanced around, and asked in alarm, "Where's Davis?" (a previous suicide attempt case). Another nurse said, "Oh that's all right, Davis is in the toilet with an orderly." Just then they both saw the orderly walking alone toward the men's ward. Both said, "My God!" and ran to the toilet, which had an open window. The patient was all right. One of the nurses explained to the observer that they had already "lost a few patients that way through the window in there."

Although both may considerably shock the staff, foreseeable and unforeseeable suicides have different impacts, particularly on nurses. Death resulting from the latter, being unprepared for and less understood, is more upsetting. As we saw in Chapter II, the distress can spread throughout other wards where people knew the patient. Yet they do not blame themselves for not having prevented the suicide—it was, after all, unforeseeable. Indeed, the staff may in such instances rationalize that if he wanted to commit suicide it was his own business. This was the general feeling about a male nurse who committed suicide because his wife was having an affair. After a post-mortem debate on balancing out what indicators they might have seen to anticipate the suicide, nurses reached the conclusion that they could not have prevented it. They felt no sense of negligence.

The response to the anticipatable suicide is not so much one of being upset at the death itself as of being upset at failure to prevent it. Staff especially accuse themselves of negligence when a patient takes his life in a known suicide space—much more, for example, than if he takes pills belonging to a nearby patient. The post-mortem debate seldom disputes the issue of anticipating the suicide, but is likely to focus on why staff did not prevent the act and how they could have. Where did they slip up? Where were they negligent? In our terms: Why did they not redefine his trajectory so that an appropriate hospital career would be instituted?

Lastly, suicide has an impact on the religious and social beliefs of nurses. It is easy enough for a nurse to justify expectable suicide without questioning her religious or social beliefs. Nurses who condemn a patient for relieving himself of great pain are seen as extreme. But when the suicide is unexpectable, nurses' religious and social beliefs may easily come into question. When nurses understand why it happens but cannot see it as justified, they are under more pressure to manage religious beliefs condemning suicide. For example, if there is an afterlife, will the suicide go to hell?

They must also confront feelings that the fault is that of "just our society" or "our hospitals." Suicide, perhaps more than other kinds of quick dying, can cause a nurse to reintegrate her beliefs about life and death with her professional position, as she tries to maintain both of them while working in terminal care.

UNEXPECTED TABLE DEATHS

A common fear of almost all adult patients who enter the operating room, even basically healthy persons going in for routine procedures, is that some unexpected factor may cause their death. And indeed, realistic as the operating staff is about these fears, they, too, may not always be completely free of similar concerns. In certain types of cases, table death is not an unrealistic expectation, but most patients do go through an operation and recover. The staff expect the large majority of patients to live, and are likely to be quite surprised at a sudden quick-dying trajectory on the operating table.

The surgeon, who knows the patient from preliminary examinations, is more likely to know in advance the possibility of trouble than are the operating room nurses, who have never seen the patient. However, the surgeon is not likely to tell them of vague suspicions (or even, sometimes, of specific suspicions) and thus leaves them unprepared for sudden death. He is likely to warn them to anticipate death only when the warning is clearly called for, as in research or high-risk surgery. Even as the operation progresses, nurses are less able than on other wards to read cues for themselves, both because they know little of the patient's record, and also because they do not always see much of his draped body on the operating table.

In spite of being in a relatively better position for anticipating trouble, doctors, too, generally expect the patient to make it through the operation, and are as completely surprised at a sudden quick dying as the nurses are. The surgeon starts the operation with a notion of what he is going to encounter, but he rarely knows with certainty. In a sense, all surgery is to some extent exploratory, and the unexpected is relatively routine. A blood vessel is in a wrong position; a person has only one kidney; an excessively enlarged heart is revealed. Any of myriad conditions can cause an emergency situation where no trouble was expected. As one operating room nurse said, "You really expect that things are going to go all right, so when they don't go all right, everybody really runs around. It gets pretty exciting." In this case, a patient hemorrhaged, which changed a rather simple operation (recovery trajectory) into a quick-dying trajectory.

When expected recovery surgery suddenly turns to quick dying, the impact on nurses varies according to the place on the ward where the dying and death occur. If the patient dies right on the table, while the operating team is doing their utmost, it is easier on the nurses than if surgery is completed and the patient dies in the recovery room. Death on the table is the end, and the staff has worked hard to prevent it. But sending the patient to the recovery room implies that he has a purchase on life; to lose this expected chance increases the surprise and shock. In the recovery room, the patient may be going back to normal fairly rapidly, and the staff are pleased with their success. If at this point a blood clot breaks off, goes to his brain, and he dies instantly, the reversal is all the more shocking because it is out of context. As one nurse said about such a pointed trajectory, "This is a real shock, it's terrible, even if you're not involved with the patient."

The kinds of surprise deaths on the table vary according to the type of hospital, the time of year, the kind of doctor, and the patient's changing condition. Hospitals vary in providing adequate facilities and skilled personnel for operations and, most important, in keeping them in practice. In major medical centers, mortality for a given operation may be zero, compared to as much as 10 per cent in hospitals that lack highly skilled surgeons and experienced nurses.[3]

3. *Time,* February, 1965.

> One of the greatest U.S. surgeons, who operates at least once a week, and on many of the world's toughest cases, has a death rate below 5%. Twelve surgeons who were technically qualified but lacked practice had a 30% death rate with less difficult cases, and one of this group lost every patient.[4]

It is no wonder that surgeons in the big centers are receiving more referrals from small cities. Mortality also varies by the month in hospitals, including big medical centers. A surgical nurse in a large medical center said, "Don't ever go into a hospital in July or August for an operation." These, of course, are the months of high turnover for nurses, interns, and residents.

Surgeons, too, vary within any one hospital, and with them varies the potential for a sudden dying trajectory. Nurses classify surgeons as "smooth" or "rough," referring to how they use their hands within the patient's body. They respect the smooth surgeon and give him their fullest support. They continually wonder how much the rough surgeon precipitates problems. He typically makes two kinds of errors of commission: one, not doing a good job, and, two, making a potentially fatal mistake, such as cutting a blood vessel or ureter and not noticing it immediately, or removing too much tissue. Although they cannot speak out, if an emergency occurs, nurses silently damn the "rough" surgeon for incompetence and dislike him intensely; sometimes they fail to meet his needs for the emergency, and the patient's fate is sealed by reciprocal antagonism between the nurses and the surgeon.

The table death clearly resulting from gross mistakes may become a coroner's case, although the doctor's status and reputation usually get him past legal difficulties. If his mistakes are infrequent, he is running on multiple good reputations for different operations, each of which is seen differently by different members of the house staff: nurses, residents, and chief surgeon. Thus, his overall reputation, mostly good, restrains potential accusations;

4. *Ibid.*

most staff "cover up" for him and are "likely to feel real bad about his error, even if the doctor is an S.O.B.," said one nurse. He goes on operating, in spite of rumors.

But if the frequency of a surgeon's table deaths exceeds some indefinable level, a single reputation develops for him, and he is less protected by staff when an issue becomes public. Moreover, staff behavior—the work order—reflects their lack of confidence. As one intern said, "I think twice now about sending a patient up for heart surgery." It was not only the patient's condition and the high-risk operating procedure that evoked caution but also the surgeon's suspect competence—this particular surgeon was himself a "high risk." [5]

Nor does having the best surgeon at the medical center insure a patient completely against errors. A top-flight surgeon is usually a teacher, and if an operation is simple he may let the resident perform some aspects of it. Thus a risk component is again introduced. "One never knows" said a post-operative nurse when asked whether a resident participated in the operation.

When an error, accident, or abrupt change in condition occurs that puts the patient into a quick dying trajectory; "everybody goes into high gear." Sometimes the sudden shift throws the gears out, and "the operating room goes to pieces." Nurses start searching their actions to see how they might have contributed to the reversal. Splendid collaboration may appear—or intense antagonism, depending, by and large, on the seeming cause of the reversal.

"The surgeon starts screaming for things and the nurse's function is to furnish them, trying to cope with the situation." As we have said, the nurse may not give the surgeon what he needs, or give it to him awkwardly if she dislikes him intensely at this moment. Sometimes the hospital does not have the right equipment for saving the patient; or the nurses, either unaware of a

---

5. To spare everyone, including patients, and the hospital image, one such surgeon was sent on an extended tour of other hospitals by the hospital administration and chief of surgery.

potential emergency that the doctor is aware of, or too inexperienced to act quickly, do not have the right tools ready at hand. Emergency turns into crisis.

When needed equipment is not at hand, the initial blame tends to fall on the surgical nurse. As one such nurse said, "Well if you don't happen to have them [instruments] there, then this is awful." The staff must work out later whether she was truly at fault. In some cases, saving may be clearly a prolonging of the patient's pain, and the rest of the team might be pleased if the right instruments for saving the patient were not readily available. But when they are not available, "commonly the doctor screams like hell at her" and the team is in crisis. The trajectory is likely to end in death, leaving the staff "shattered," unable to pinpoint anybody with the blame for missing the chance to save the patient.

Reinstating a satisfactory sentimental order after a sudden quick-dying trajectory and an operating table death involves several factors. One lies in the self-selective recruitment of operating room nurses. By and large, nurses who wish to be on an operating room team are considerably and basically more involved with the surgeon than with the patients. They idolize doctors; they want to help them as collaborators; they want contact with doctors. During the operation their focus is on helping the doctor and meeting the test it puts them through. Indeed, many operating room nurses find the operating room "a marvelous way to get away from the patient." When setting up instruments for an emergency, they are preparing to aid the doctor more than preparing for a table death. Thus, with sudden dying, the sentimental order is all the more shattered for a nurse who cannot aid the doctor because of not having the right instruments. Conversely, the doctor can do a great deal to restore that order by indicating that he does not blame the nurse for lack of preparation.

If nurses are prepared for an emergency but the patient still suddenly dies, the key to maintaining or regaining their composure often lies in their strong feelings toward the doctor. It is usually compassion for his misfortune. Generated by their strong involvement with him, their compassion focuses on *his* involvement with the patient.

The nurses' lack of involvement with the particular patient and his trajectory is facilitated by several barriers that separate the patient from them. They usually do not see the patient until he is on the table, and then only see a part of his body. Only in small towns and/or in small hospitals is it likely that the OR nurses know of the patient as a person. In larger hospitals, there are many people around—aides, students, etc.—to dilute any occasion that might involve an OR nurse with the patient. The OR nurses' job on the team also affects her possible involvement. If she is the scrub nurse, she is very busy handing instruments to the doctor. The circulating nurse is liable to some involvement with the patient because her job allows time to squeeze in a little talk with him. This contact is especially motivated by individual disposition; it is not part of her job.

The nature of operating room work also creates a barrier between nurse and patient. It is very intense and precise, requiring nurses "to be strong at all costs." Sentiments are not allowed to interfere with the precision of the work order. The work pace forces them to get used to all contingencies of surgery, including sights, smells and sudden dying.

As we have noted earlier, barriers that reduce nurses' involvement with the patient also reduce the depth of their feelings about a sudden quick dying trajectory and death. The sentimental order that is not touched too deeply is relatively easily preserved or restored. To be sure, for some nurses the distress is great and may prompt an extreme disruption of the work order. One nurse, discussing such a situation, admitted, "I left the operating room because I couldn't stand it any longer."

To help reinstate the sentimental order for nurses, some physicians will turn a patient who suddenly starts to die on the table over to a "special nurse" who takes over his care in the recovery room. This minimizes the OR nurses' involvement in the dying by "*deflecting* from this tremendous reality that someone is dying right there . . . people [staff] act as though it's really not going on, yet there it is." The nurses on the operating team do not have to talk of the dying nor do anything to avert it, which helps to reinstate the sentimental order. Such story-making as they may engage in is based on brief medical reports on the patient's condition, not on their own participation in the ordeal.

In spite of structural barriers to involvement, some aspects of a quick-dying surgery patient may disturb the nurses very much. One is social loss. During table talk of an operation, nurses may hear someone say, "So this is a woman with three kids." If the patient suddenly starts to die, her social loss is very upsetting. Children and young adults also imply severe social loss that upsets the nurses. A dying VIP also may touch the nurses if they realize who he is. The reinstatement of sentimental order disrupted by social loss is handled by "loss rationales," which we have written about at length elsewhere.[6] Briefly, nurses fashion these rationales to explain to each other why it is better in the long run that the patient died.

Another aspect of involvement is the dying or death rehearsal that the patient provides for the nurses. Patients in the same age group as a nurse, or with a similar condition, have this effect. Also, witnessing a condition that might happen to them—a breast removal, for example—which ends in a quick dying trajectory is shocking for the nurses. The sentimental order in these cases is reinstated by the nurses' personally working through their own possible fate, with the aid and support of their fellow nurses who have come to terms with these possibilities for themselves.

The new operating room nurse or students may become paralyzed at the sight of a sudden quick dying trajectory. The presence of these people in turn can obstruct the performance of the remainder of the staff. The interruption of the sentimental and work order of the team is handled by getting the neophyte out of the room: "Well, the staff doesn't like to have this kind of a mess

6. Glaser and Strauss, "Social Loss of Dying Patients," *American Journal of Nursing,* Vol. 64 (June, 1964), pp. 119–21.

to handle. You have enough problems around without some weak-kneed kid to handle." The inexperienced nurse who breaks down or paralyzes breaks the rule of being strong at all costs, a rule that is a partial foundation of the work and sentimental order. Experienced nurses, when upset at changes in trajectory, at least are practiced in putting up a front of composure.

VIII

Last Weeks and Days

Unless a person dies abruptly, with virtually no warning, the dying trajectory includes a stage of "last days" and perhaps even "last weeks." The hospital staff responsible for his care usually finds itself engaged in a complex juggling of tasks, people, and relationships. Analysis of that juggling is the principal aim of this chapter. Because of its complexity, we cannot fully detail the myriad variants that arise, but a schematic treatment should be sufficient to carry the dying trajectory forward to its next phase, the hours just prior to death, and then to the death scene itself.

JUGGLING

The staff's juggling consists, first, of organizing a number of potentially shifting treatment and care tasks. As a patient becomes visibly sicker and weaker, the staff typically stop certain activities and simultaneously initiate new ones. The comfort care activities may become very detailed and may now require considerable nursing skill; the medical care necessary to keep him alive may remain quite complex, although different from earlier medical care.

Meanwhile, the staff must also juggle people and relationships whose existence can cause great disruption to the ward's work and sentimental orders. If the patient is visible to other patients, their reactions to his last weeks and days must be taken into account, particularly insofar as they may see his dying as a rehearsal of their own. The problems of family management also are potentially great. Family members must be warned about the oncoming death, prepared for it, perhaps given occasional emotional support, and warned against bringing the patient into awareness if it is undesirable for him to know about his approaching death. The patient himself, unless he is virtually comatose, also represents a range of potential problems for the staff. He may not die acceptably, according to ward standards; may not come to terms with his dying; may ask uncomfortable questions, even if he is not aware of his oncoming death. Like the treatment and care tasks, the management of people and relationships shifts as the trajectory moves along. Whenever their handling of such work is inadequate, both the staff's work and the accompanying collective moods are profoundly affected. Things are, so to speak, out of order.

STRUCTURAL RELEVANCES

The range of potential problems a staff faces is measurably reduced by the systematic routing of dying patients into the appropriate wards of a hospital. Each ward, as we noted in Chapter III, tends to have its own limited range of probable dying trajectories, with personnel geared to coping with various phases of those trajectories. When unusual trajectories occur on a ward, the personnel are far less prepared to cope with either the medical treatment or the social-psychological aspects of the last days. They may not even anticipate various social-psychological problems that accompany those last days.

For the usual trajectories, however, the ward possesses considerable resources of skill, organization, and perhaps equipment, which can be brought into play when warranted. In short, the ward's structure is adaptable to specified phases of its typical trajectories. This structural adaptability is also found, as we shall suggest later, on the large, all-purpose, and therefore infinitely multitrajectoried wards characteristically found in countries outside Western Europe and North America. But although the structural resources of each ward are brought into play at appropriate moments, our familiar key variables (awareness, social loss, etc.) are also likely to affect whether and how this is done.

TEMPORAL ORDER AND CRITICAL JUNCTURES

Despite the institutional mechanisms for standardizing trajectories and the structural resources available for dealing with them,
the organization of work is constantly in delicate balance. So much
can go wrong: so much is unexpected. This would be true even
if dying were "timeless" or took place only over a short period.
But last days take time; hospital personnel must juggle tasks,
people, and relationships that can and do change daily. And the
three orders of changes affect one another. This is why we
earlier emphasized that the total organization of activity (which
we call work) during the course of dying is profoundly affected
by temporal considerations. We referred to the entire web of
such relationships on a ward as its temporal order. This order
includes the continual readjustment and coordination of staff
effort.

Temporal order is threatened by a whole host of changes,
which we shall detail below, and considerable staff activity during
the patient's last days is likely to be directed at maintaining a workable temporal order. Since every ward has many patients, usually
including some who are not dying, the entire matter is rendered
all the more complicated than if the staff needed only to balance
one patient, his "kin" and its own involvement.

One final point before we turn to detailed discussion of the
last days: As we have seen, there is much variation in the duration
and shape of trajectories. Among trajectories that do include
recognizable last weeks or days, three major classes are especially
important. The first is when death is uncertain but, if it occurs, is
quick. The second type is when death is certain but the time of
death is relatively uncertain; the patient may linger with reprieves,
plateaus, and even partial reversals. The third type is when both
death and time of death are relatively certain. Each type tends
to involve the staff in a somewhat different range of problems with
patient, family, and neighboring patients. Each type also gives
rise to somewhat different strategies for handling various critical

junctures—defining a patient as in his last weeks or days, pre-announcing his probable death, "deciding" whether to prolong or hasten his dying, and engaging in and arranging for farewells and last looks. Such critical junctures may be only episodes during the last phases of the trajectory, or they may be turning points in the final evolution of a dying patient's trajectory. Moreover, a given critical juncture may appear more than once, and repetition itself alters the character of the juncture and may raise special problems.

FAMILY HANDLING

Major Problems

Most patients belong to families. If kinsmen appear at the bedside of a dying relative during last days, their presence can pose severe problems for the medical and nursing personnel, and may actually interfere with the efficient care of patients. Problems tend to center around four issues: the family needs to be prepared for the forthcoming death; they may need to be persuaded to delegate responsibility for the dying person to the hospital; they may require coaching in proper modes of behavior while at the hospital; and they may need to be helped in their grieving, either for their own sake or for the sake of preventing disruption of ward activity. The nature of these central problems suggests that the personnel may be considerably engaged in working with the family during the last days.

Sometimes work with families is unnecessary or minimal. If there is no family or none close enough to visit the hospital, no family problems arise. In American geriatric hospitals, for example, family-handling problems are minimal. Many families never visit, either because they live too far away or because they have already abandoned the patient. Often kinsmen arrive at the hospital only at the very point of death; if they visit earlier, their visits tends to be short and infrequent. Since the dying relative is elderly and perhaps has been dying for a long time, visitors are likely to grieve but little, and quietly. In a ward populated largely by senile and comatose patients, these intrusions have minimal effects.

In some countries, especially in economically underdeveloped areas, close kinsmen customarily provide the comfort care to dying relatives, thus relieving nursing personnel for other duties. In these hospitals, moreover, families often provide feeding, bathing, and general routine care to recovering patients, so staff are accustomed to their presence. Grieving kinsmen tend to support one another, and when several work around one patient they may grieve collectively.

In striking contrast are those conditions that tend to maximize disruption of the staff's work and the ward's atmosphere. At a small hospital in Gubbio, Italy, we witnessed the following drama. Just as we entered the ward, a daughter ran out of her dying father's room, screaming loudly for a doctor: "My father is dying!" Other patients and their kinsmen quickly gathered and stared at the developing scene. Two nurses also quickly appeared, then scampered into the dying man's room, closing the door behind them. In the hall the distraught daughter was comforted by her husband. A few moments later, a physician scurried down the corridor, entered the room, and soon came out and told the excited couple nothing could be done for the old man, that he only had a few days to live. Then he left them, returning to his interrupted work. In cases like this, the family often spirits their relative away from the hospital, wishing him to die at home—and thus inevitably hastening his death. But if he does not die within a day or two, they may bring him back to the hospital, thinking he may be saved, not recognizing he has only had a reprieve.

As we have seen, unexpected death can cause the family to act drastically toward the physician or nurses. If a family is to be prepared for a patient's death, it must be forewarned. The physician is responsible for disclosing probable death. His timing depends on many variables. Chief among them is the nature of the expected dying trajectory. If, for example, surgery can—perhaps—give a few extra years of life, but only at great risk, then parents customarily are told that their child may not survive the operation. If a patient suffers a stroke, is brought to the hospital, and is judged to have only a few remaining days or weeks, then, too, the family is likely to be warned of the virtual certainty of death. On the other hand, extensively lingering trajectories allow the physician great latitude in timing his preannouncements to the family. Indeed, he does not know exactly when the patient will die and may not be able to predict whether there will be temporary reprieves, plateaus, and even reversals. His first preannouncement of death may be long delayed, or consist initially of cues to which the family can respond with gradually growing awareness. He may make several preannouncements during the last weeks and days, indicating that death is getting closer.

Some physicians develop considerable skill at pacing out these preannouncements. Ineffective pacing—or insufficient trust by the family—may result in their shopping around for a "better" doctor, one with a cure, even though cure is really not at issue. Good strategy usually requires that the physician make his first preannouncement to the "strongest" family member, who then has the responsibility of disclosing this (and subsequent) information to other relatives as he judges they can take it.

During the last days, family members may ply the hospital staff with queries bearing not only on time (how many days, hours, has he got to live?) but also on mode of dying (will he die peacefully, will he be entirely out of pain?). Those queries must be handled. If they are not, scenes are likely to erupt on the ward.[1]

Some families have sufficient internal resources for accepting the forthcoming death of a relative, but sometimes the staff finds it necessary to help them come to terms with the event. The staff then offers them loss rationales or supports those created by the kinsmen: "Yes, it will be a blessing if he goes soon." "Yes, he's lucky that he has no pain at all." If the last days stretch into last weeks, the staff can sustain the relatives' acceptance by displaying equanimity and by giving undiminished comfort care to the pa-

1. For fuller discussion of preannouncement strategies and problems, see *Awareness of Dying, op. cit.*

tient. (They may even act out a drama like that portrayed in the previous chapter when the husband would not "give up" on his wife.) The staff can give assurances that the patient will die peacefully. They can correct unfounded expectations concerning his mode of dying. When plateaus or reprieves occur, staff can show pleasure without encouraging false hopes, signaling quietly that death is still on the way. If need be, the nurses can put pressure on the physician to "explain again" to a close relative who will not really face the facts. On one pediatric ward, we observed a staff discussion in which nurses pressured the resident to make a mother "begin grieving," make her "really realize" that her child was not going to recover. On this ward, it is a standard tactic to get the grieving started long before the anticipated death.

Relatives' acceptance of a forthcoming death is likely to be linked with whether they have already partly gotten over their grief or have at least gotten it under control. By the last days of an extremely slow trajectory, virtually everybody may be fairly well "grieved out," especially if the patient's social loss is relatively low. Occasionally a latecomer arrives who has only recently heard the news, and who displays his grief; this in turn may prompt other kinsmen to renew their grieving, or to put on an act in which they show more grief than they really now feel, or to explain that they are all worn out and past his stage of grieving.

If at all possible, a tactful staff allows close kinsmen plenty of time with the dying person, especially during the very last days, so that they can quietly live through their grieving. Sometimes personnel do not recognize the grieving as such—it has many individual and cultural variants. But by and large they do understand that a wife must be with a dying husband, children with a dying parent, that separation would be more painful than "participation" in the dying. Some hospitals have convenient rooms where relatives may wait when they cannot stay at the bedside. At one Scottish hospital, staff members offer the relatives "spirits" and overt consolation; in American hospitals, sedatives are more likely to accompany the consolation.

When the family or the staff believes it advisable that the dying person remain ignorant of his forthcoming death, family members must take care not to display their grief before the patient. Staff members may have to warn kinsmen about this danger or take steps to prevent its occurrence. Since grieving may begin the instant that close kinsmen are told about the probability of death, the staff may immediately begin giving support. In one Greek hospital that we visited, this supportive tactic was highly institutionalized: the head of the nursing service customarily made the preannouncement in her office and then supported the stunned kinsmen.

As we have noted, nursing personnel often find their role as sympathetic listener or comforter a major one during the final days. They are especially empathetic when they regard the patient's death as a grave social loss, or when their compassion is especially aroused by an association with their own personal past, or, sometimes, when a grieving family member has behaved admirably in the face of the ordeal. Occasionally a mother has lost another child, or perhaps a sister, from the same hereditary disease; the social-loss aspect adds both to the mother's grief and to the staff's efforts to console her.

In American hospitals, social workers tend self-consciously to become "grief-workers," attempting with professional deliberateness to "work through" the grief of relatives; this is perhaps most noticeable on pediatric wards. Priests, chaplains, and nuns also engage in such activities; indeed, they may be called on by a desperate nursing staff afraid of the disastrous effects of death and unable themselves to help the relative. We have observed a chaplain intervene during the last days in a situation of growing animosity between staff and a wife whose unacceptable behavior apparently was due to her failure to come to terms with her husband's oncoming death. In American hospitals, psychiatrists may also be called in to work with family members.

The staff's third problem of family handling—getting suitable behavior from the family members—is linked closely with whether the family is adequately prepared for the death, and does its

grieving "on schedule." As we have seen, a wife may cause upsetting scenes if she is not at all prepared for her husband's death
when it finally draws near. A relative who grieves too early and
openly may disturb the patient; even if the latter is quite aware
of his forthcoming death, he may not yet be sufficiently resigned
to it.

The staff may also have to coach relatives in appropriate bedside behavior. If family members visit in too great numbers, a
rule may be laid down that only close kin can visit "from now
on"—especially as death becomes imminent. A family that is too
noisy may need to be reprimanded; the staff may forbid access
to the ward to all but the closest kin. Once we observed the
nurses intervene in a situation in which a lower income family
noisily "carried on right in the room as if the patient were not
dying"; the physician was prevailed upon to allow only the mother
and father visiting rights to the bedside.

On large, open wards, visitors must be especially careful not
to disturb nearby patients with chattering or loud sobbing, even
when they and the dying man are hidden behind a screen. When
the patient has a private room, kin still may need to be taught
not to "get in the way." Often a nurse will ask someone to leave
the bedside or the room when she suspects that a nursing or medical procedure may disturb the onlooker. Visitors may also harass
the staff by making what the latter considers unjustified, over-
anxious, or just plain fussy demands. Various tactics are used to
make the offending person behave properly or, if that proves impossible, to avoid contact with the person as much as possible.
What is considered unjustified or fussy depends not only on the
behavior itself, but also on how attached the personnel have become to the patient, how well they have come to know the family member, the nature of the patient's evolving story, and so on.
The staff may call on other family members to restrain the over-
demanding person. It may also rely on kinsmen to restrain each
other's improper use of space and to control each other's noisi-
ness, as well as to help each other to grieve on schedule, and to

make judgments about who should not visit the hospital or how close the patient is to his final moments.

The staff's fourth great problem is that the kinsmen may not willingly delegate the patient's care during his last hours. Unwillingness to delegate may vary in seriousness. At its most extreme, the patient simply is withdrawn from the hospital, usually against professional advice. He may even literally be kidnapped before the staff is quite aware of what has happened (or so we have been told by nurses at foreign hospitals). Unwillingness to leave a patient in the hospital during his last hours may derive from the family's fear that he will die there rather than at home, where they feel he belongs. But their unwillingness may also be associated (as with Malayan villagers) with religious practices that they know cannot be carried out within the hospital. Sometimes an American family takes a patient home during his last days because it believes it can provide adequate care there; the family may discover its error later and return him to the hospital.

Even families who know very well that their dying kinsman should remain in professional hands may try to interfere with the staff, suggesting or demanding that certain things be done differently. The staff require countertactics to cope with this behavior. More generally, however, the division of labor in American hospitals allows close kin to carry out routine comfort care while the nursing staff gives the more difficult or professionalized care. As the last days draw to a close, sometimes the staff tactfully allows a mother or wife to take over the comfort care almost totally if the mode of dying permits such latitude. Nurses may sense that the active kinsman needs to give this care; she would suffer more from inactivity. In many Asian and European hospitals it is standard practice to leave to family members almost complete responsibility for the comfort care of dying relatives. In a Japanese hospital, for instance, we talked with a patient dying of cancer, whose mother had accompanied him to Tokyo from a distant northern region in order to care for him during his last weeks and days. At this hospital, such an arrangement was usual.

STRUCTURAL CONDITIONS

Neither the severity of problems that a family will present the hospital staff nor the degree of success the staff will have in managing a family during the last weeks and days are entirely predictable. Yet it is possible to state in general terms the kinds of structural conditions that militate against the relative tranquillity and success of the staff's efforts at management. Among those conditions are the number of visiting relatives, the distance from which they come, the experience they have with hospital customs and rules, the amount of trust they have in the professionals, and the amount or kind of ward space.

An especially important structural condition is created by the combination of type of dying trajectory and type of ward. We see the impact of this conjuncture clearly in the ICU, where a fair proportion of patients are likely to be in their last days, sometimes with rather short warning to relatives. Space limitations and the intensive character of staff work, plus the maximum visibility of patients to each other, make it necessary to keep bedside visiting very brief. Nurses develop special tactics for gentling the relatives out the door and for avoiding the pleading faces of relatives sitting restlessly in the nearby waiting room.

Prior to severe surgery or when an emergency operation is in progress—a touch-and-go situation with a strong potential of last days or last hours—family members tend to wander from the surgery waiting room to the nursing station, bombarding personnel with anxious queries and expressive chatter. Although personnel have developed standard tactics for handling families, these tactics are not always successful in these conditions. With unexpectedly quick or potentially nonrecoverable trajectories, for example, the family's queries may have to be evaded until the trajectory is more certain or until the physician can disclose it to the family. [We remember vividly how an extensive Gypsy family swarmed over a ward during an emergency operation on a kinsman. The family gave the staff a very difficult time. There were not enough staff members, and not enough time was available, to permit efficient use of the standard tactics evolved for handling more normal sized and more "disciplined" families.]

Even in such trying situations, however, a staff can sometimes count or call on some other family member to exert a controlling hand. Staff members can also draw on various resources of the ward: the telephone may call them away; they can set up spatial barriers to keep a family at arm's length; they can escape by throwing themselves with obvious gestures into their work; if need be, they can invoke rarely used hospital rules. The staff may even turn to the families of other patients, who sometimes can be counted on to help restrain or reassure an upset family.

We should not think of the structural conditions, which lessen or enlarge problems of family handling, as static. If they were, the staff's control would, paradoxically, be rendered both more difficult and much easier. The longer a lingering trajectory is, the more structural conditions are likely to change; some changes help the staff, some hinder it. Indeed, many of the most disturbing events stem from evolving conditions so unusual that the staff does not anticipate them, and may not be able to do much to prevent their recurrence. Handling the immediate situation necessitates that the staff grasp an unusual structural condition.

Here are a few examples of such conditions: first, a structural condition that is expected to change but does not. When a hospitalized child dies over a period of months, the staff ordinarily expects the parents to become more prepared for the death. But in a Rome hospital, nurses told us of parents who caused upsetting scenes during their child's last days because they could not believe he was dying, even though he had been hospitalized a year before with a diagnosis of certain death. The same hospital provides an example of an unanticipated structural condition and its consequences: The nursing personnel claim to have special difficulties with southern Italians, who are "more expressive" in their grieving and who are not familiar with proper standards of behavior in hospitals. They press for long visiting hours and for visits at inappropriate times. The standard tactics that nurses employ to control such families sometimes break down when the responsible staff physician also happens to be southern Italian; rather than becoming their ally, he may actually allow the offending family special license to visit as they wish. The nurses must then devise new tactics to handle the family.

In a Scottish hospital, by contrast, an overly expressive Italian family's visits and visiting time were cut down because of its noise, in order to minimize further disturbance of the ward. In another Scottish hospital, a nurse described how one family's queries about their kinsman's condition were enormously difficult to handle because the patient happened to be her own uncle—a structural condition that remained relatively out of her control during the entire course of his dying.

Occasionally, a responsible family member may distress the staff not by what he does but rather by what he does not do. When, for example, a wife begins to visit her dying husband less and less frequently, the staff may be sufficiently disturbed to ask the staff physician or the chaplain to intervene, either to discover "what's wrong" or to urge more attention by the wife.

LEAVE-TAKING

As the last weeks move into last days, and the last days into probable last hours, a critical juncture arises that can be particularly hazardous for the work and sentiments of personnel. That juncture comes when close relatives say final (or tentatively final) farewells to the dying patient or—if he is not aware—when they take their last looks at him while he still lives. Told through a preannouncement that he has not long to live, or warned by their own senses, they take leave silently or openly.

These leave-takings are likely to be awesome ceremonies, even when the dying man is comatose, has been socially dead for some time, or is elderly. Each day's separation implies the possibility that *this* may be the last time visitors will see the patient alive. When family members travel considerable distances to visit at the hospital, as is characteristic at regional hospitals and metropolitan medical centers, they may be able to visit only on weekends or at intervals of at least several days. They must make each farewell not knowing whether they will return before their relative has died.

The anguish of visitors' farewells may be shared by some staff members. We saw this in the dying of a lovely teenaged girl who lingered long. Her mother visited each day, and stayed all day. The staff members became as attached to the mother as to the daughter. When the dying continued to stretch out over many days, each one possibly the girl's last, the collective mood of the staff grew increasingly tense. Each night when the mother left for home staff members felt—and some showed—great empathetic anxiety. Eventually, a solution to the daily leave-taking was found. Since the mother was a practical nurse, possessing sufficient skills to care for her daughter at home if given proper equipment and instruction, the nursing staff negotiated with the physician; and together they agreed that the mother, who increasingly wished to have her daughter spend her last days at home, should be allowed her wish. After that decision was implemented, the entire staff breathed more freely, but its tension took a few days to dissipate. The most important immediate change was that the ward's normal temporal order, which had been disrupted by time spent with the mother or daughter and by time spent talking about one or another of them, was reestablished. On wards where "final" leave-takings are frequent and anguished, the disruption of temporal work and sentimental orders is sometimes devastating.

MANAGING THE PATIENT'S TRAJECTORY

During his last weeks and days, the patient is much more likely than his family to be the center of the staff's attention, unless he is comatose, scarcely sentient, or so ill as hardly to be reacting as a person. Under these latter conditions, the staff's juggling of its tasks, around him and around its relationships with him, need only be minimal. Major problems, however, are set for the personnel when the patient's expected last days stretch out interminably on wards organized for faster turnover of patients, or when a patient's mode of dying is so extraordinarily unpleasant as to disturb staff members.

If the dying person is sentient but unaware of his impending death, then the staff's major problems may be associated with keeping him unaware, or at least keeping his suspicions sufficiently damped down so that his trajectory can be shaped as seems wise.[2] If his pain is so great that the staff can stand neither his physical anguish nor his obviously increasing awareness of his waning life, the patient can be "snowed" with drugs during his final days. We shall look now at only a few of the major problems faced by staff, or family, or the patient himself during his last days.

If the patient has become aware that he is dying, through direct or indirect preannouncement, or through his reading of staff's behavioral cues and his own symptoms, his awareness necessitates his coming to terms with dying. If by virtue of a slow trajectory he has had many months to face his mortality, he has probably entered or reentered the hospital better prepared than if his period of awareness has been short or sudden. If he is not elderly and has not already come to terms with advanced age (or even with death), a quick trajectory is likely to precipitate crises of awareness for the sentient patient, as well as for his family. Such crises affect the management of his trajectory.

Even in slow dying, the breakthrough of awareness during last days can be traumatic. The staff sometimes has little control over the structural conditions that determine the impact. For instance, a patient may know he has an extremely serious illness, but not regard it as fatal. The preannouncement suddenly is made to him, or a disclosure is made inadvertently. We observed, for example, the last days of a teenager who had learned of his imminent death from a friend who had learned of it from another friend, whose parents in turn had received the information from the patient's parents. The blinding news, combined with a deep sense of his parents' betrayal, resulted, as staff members put it, in the boy's

2. For fuller discussion, see *Awareness of Dying, op. cit.*

almost complete "withdrawal" and "apathy." Consequently, the staff could do almost nothing to shape his trajectory as they would have wished. Even the psychiatrist whom they called in could accomplish nothing.

During the hospitalization of another patient, however, the personnel were partly responsible for creating a structural condition that genuinely prevented their shaping of her trajectory. This woman, who was lingering in great pain, was far less afraid of death than of dying with uncontrollable pain. She had good reason for her fear, for she did not trust the nursing staff to control her pain, much less prevent its increase. The house physician in charge was desperate both because he could not control her growing pain and because he was in the crossfire from his patient, who respected him, and the nurses, who wished him to discipline her complaining. Finally, aware that she was dying, the patient allowed him to arrange an operation that might lessen her pain, although it was not likely to have any direct bearing on the course of her illness. She permitted the operation although she was intensely afraid that it would leave her "a vegetable." This woman's complaints about tardy and ineffective medication for her pain, her fear of dying in pain, her indecision over whether to permit the final operation (she died during surgery)—all conspired to rock the house staff, to cause considerable strain between nurses and the house physician, and to prevent the staff from shaping her trajectory.

THE MEANING OF DEATH

On the other hand, a slow trajectory often gives the patient opportunities to come to terms with his own mortality, for his awareness and understanding may develop sufficiently early so that he can confront his dying. Such coming to terms involves two separate processes. The first consists of facing the annihilation of self, of visualizing a world without one's self. The second process consists of facing up to dying as a physical, and perhaps mental, disintegration. Some people are fearful of dying in great pain, or with extreme bodily disfiguration or with loss of speech, or are perhaps afraid of "just lying there like a vegetable." Some people think hardly at all about these aspects of dying, but tremble at the prospect of the disappearance of self. Moreover, some patients who have come to terms with the idea of death may only later focus on dying, especially when, as the trajectory advances, they are surprised, dismayed, or otherwise affected by bodily changes. On the other hand, someone who lives with his dying long enough may become assured that he will "pass" peacefully enough, and only then fully face the death issue.

These two issues, which generally loom large during the last sentient days, are certainly not unrelated; nor does coming to terms with them always constitute a final settlement. Unexpected turns in the trajectory are likely to unsettle previous preparations. With unexpected bodily deterioration, patients panic or begin to lose recognition of themselves as known identities. In one instance of great insight, a patient told a nurse she feared "comfort" surgery would cause her to "die twice." It might help to relieve her pain for a period, but eventually she would have to face dying again.

Most frequently, perhaps, patients come to terms by themselves or with the participation of close kin. Nurses, however, may be drawn into the processes. The patient typically initiates the "death talk"; the nurse tends to listen, to assent, to be sympathetic, to reassure. The nurse may even cry with a patient. Occasionally, a patient repeatedly invites nurses into conversations about death or dying, but they decline his invitations. Their refusals tend to initiate a drama of mutual pretense: neither party subsequently indicates recognition of the forthcoming death, although both know about it.

Other parties, too, sometimes play significant roles in these processes. In one such situation, an elderly patient was rescued from the isolation of mutual pretense by a hospital chaplain who directly participated in his coming to terms; eventually he also persuaded the wife, and to some extent the nurses, to enter into the continuing conversation. Patients sometimes rely on members of the clergy to move their spouses to faster acceptance of the inevitable and thus ease their own acceptance.

On the whole, American nurses seem to find it difficult to carry on conversations about death or dying with patients. Only if a patient has already come to terms with death, or if they can honestly assure him he will die "easily," if he is elderly, do they find it relatively easy to talk about such topics with him.[3] Unless a patient shows considerable composure about his dying, nurses and physicians lose their composure, except when they are specially trained or specially suited by temperament, or have some unusual empathy with a patient because of a similarity of personal history. When the patient's conversation during the last days is only obliquely about death and dying—consisting, for instance, of reminiscences of the past—and is not unpleasant or unduly repetitious, he has a better chance of inducing others, including the nurses, to participate in his closing of his life.

Clergymen also are expected, in most countries, to play major roles in this phasing-out of patients. A dying Greek patient who belonged to the Coptic faith completely upset the machinery of a Greek hospital by insisting late at night that he needed a Coptic priest immediately to give him his final communion. The request was almost impossible to fulfill at that hour, but the staff felt obliged to do so. A priest was found, but only just in time. In the United States, psychiatrists also sometimes perform analogous functions during the last phasing-out of more secularized patients.[4]

TYING UP LOOSE ENDS

An important aspect of a patient's coming to terms with impending death is the closing off of various aspects of everyday business. These include material and personal matters, like the drawing-up of wills and the making-up of quarrels. Physicians

---

3. Jeanne C. Quint, *The Nurse and the Dying Patient* (New York: Macmillan, 1967); "Mastectomy—Symbol of Cure or Warning Sign?", *GP*, XXIX (March, 1964), pp. 119–24; "The Impact of Mastectomy," *The American Journal of Nursing*, 63 (November, 1963), pp. 88–92.
4. Personal communications from several psychiatrists.

seem apt to allow businessmen to close off their business dealings, though a patient may have to insist on his right to do so, and to permit distraught families to urge reluctant patients to draw up, alter, or sign wills. A lawyer is sometimes brought in by the family or physician to help persuade the patient to make or alter his will. A chaplain or priest sometimes considers that his professional duties include bridging relationships between the dying person and an alienated spouse or offspring. One chaplain elatedly described how he had been instrumental in bringing a patient, her husband, her parents, and her children to face death together. This patient had gone ahead of her kinsmen in facing her death, and could no longer really talk with them. The chaplain bridged over the awkward relationships.

Sometimes the patient accepts his forthcoming death even before the staff has quite come to terms with it. Moreover, the patient's "social willing" may shock his family or the staff precisely because he has imaginatively reached his life's end before they have. One patient, for instance, relied on the intervention of his sister (who happened to be a nurse) to will his library to a neighboring college; his wife would never discuss the matter with him. A more extreme instance of social willing, which shocked personnel, was when a patient, during his last days, insisted on signing his own autopsy papers. This action struck the staff as singularly grotesque, despite the accepted similar practice of willing one's eyes, brain, or entire body to hospitals.

TEMPORAL INCONGRUITIES

Still another great barrier may block even the best-intentioned nurses and physicians from providing adequate help to a patient when he faces his demise: the immense difference between the staff's and the patient's conceptions of time. As we have noted repeatedly, the staff operates on "work time." Their tasks are guided by schedules, which on most wards are related to many patients, both dying and recovering. More important, and more subtle, work time with a given dying patient is a matter of timing work according to his expected trajectory. He is supposed to die more or less "on time," even when that time is uncertain. Our data, as well as accounts by dying patients or by kin who have participated intimately in relatives' dying, suggest that a patient's personal sense of time, undergoes striking changes once he becomes aware of his impending death. This occurs whether he becomes aware very early or very late.

The last days become structured in highly personalized temporal terms. The future is foreshortened, cut out, or abstracted to "after I am gone." The personal past is likely to be reviewed and reconceptualized. The present takes on various kinds of personal meanings. Author Bernice Kavinovsky noted, for example: "All week, although I teach my classes, arrange for a substitute, put the dinner on, telephone my son at his apartment, shower, mark manuscripts, I perform each act almost clinically aware of the obstruction in my breast." She was "at the same time assailed on every hand by beauty's endless argument—an arc of light, or the curve of my husband's cheek . . . or the noise of the children's games on the roof next door"—the sights and sounds of the world taking on sudden and astonishing beauty.[5] Various semi-mystical experiences may be associated with the new temporal references. Things previously taken for granted are now savored as unique but unfortunately transitory. Occasional reprieves, recognized as only reprieves, evoke temporally significant reactions running from, "Oh, God! take me, I was prepared and now will not be prepared" to gratefulness for unexpected time.

The important point is not so much the variability of temporal reconstructions as the difficulty, and sometimes complete inability, of outsiders to grasp these personal reconstructions. One cannot know about them unless privy to the dying person's thoughts. He may keep them to himself, especially in a context of mutual pretense. He may not be able to express them clearly, especially when he becomes less sentient. A busy staff may have little time to listen or to invite revealing talk, particularly if pa-

5. *Voyage and Return: An Experience with Cancer* (New York: W. W. Norton, 1966), p. 20.

tients are competing for attention. In many American hospitals nursing aides spend more time in patients' rooms than the nurses do, even during last days. When aides manage to grasp a patient's temporal reordering of his life, they may be unable to pass along this knowledge to the nurses, or not feel free to do so, or assume that the information is unimportant.

When the patient's personal time and the staff's work time are highly disparate, considerable strain may be engendered. Nor is the source of the trouble necessarily evident to either. Sometimes, of course, the staff does sense something of a patient's reconceptualizations, without necessarily realizing their deep import, and may somewhat adjust its own work time to his requirements. Thus on a medical ward housing many cancer patients, which we studied, there was a ward ideology of "letting them set the pace," with work time considerably structured around the patients' relatively slow tempo. Within limits, cancer patients could negotiate, for instance, to eat or have their temperatures taken later than when ordinarily scheduled.

ISOLATION

A staff's failure to understand a patient's attempts at achieving psychological closure in his life contributes to another process: the patient's increasing isolation, whether or not he perceives it. He may, of course, understand very well that staff members are not interested in his awesome problem, or cannot grasp its nature even if they wish to. If he has tried to communicate with the staff, he may despair of their understanding. Or he may prefer to communicate with his family or his minister, although he may actually be unable to "reach" them either.[6]

However, it is not only the communications problem that produces isolation. In all the countries where we have observed, we found strong tendencies to start isolating a dying patient during his last days in the hospital. Isolation techniques—perhaps "insulation" is a better term—have their source in various structural

6. Cf. Jeanne Quint, *op. cit,* "The Impact. . . ."

conditions. For instance, if everyone agrees that a patient should be kept unaware, then attempts to buffer him from knowledge immediately set in motion a train of insulating mechanisms.[7] The isolating process is also called into play if the patient is aware but accepts or invites mutual pretense about his dying. The isolating mechanisms are blunted, however, if the patient is openly aware; even then, staff may begin to avoid death talk or even the patient's room.

The patient who will not accept his dying or is dying in a socially unacceptable way also arouses avoidance—sometimes by his family as well as the staff. One of the clearest examples of this that we saw was an ICU nurse's brusque handling of a quite sentient patient who looked only a few hours away from death. The nurse described him as "ornery"; in brief, he was "asking for it." Personnel on the medical ward from which this dying man had been transferred had also regarded him as difficult and unreasonable.

During a patient's last days, the staff lightens its work and increases the probability of giving good comfort care by moving him closer to the nursing station. Of course, he may be grateful for the added security of being near the staff, but the move may frighten him despite the nurses' explanations. And in large wards, the move not only tells the aware patient that he is nearing his end, but it also may isolate him from satisfying friendships he has made with other patients. Because of unpleasant odors or perhaps uncontrollable groans and sobbing, he may even be moved into a separate room, or may be shielded from the ward by a temporary screen. This is sometimes done even before the last hours, especially if he is judged disturbing to other patients. In hospitals where patients are housed in smaller rooms, the staff tends during the last days to put the dying patient either into a single room or with a comatose patient. If the roommate is not comatose, he may complain about the dying patient's behavior, and this stimulates the staff to move one or the other. Of course, when patients

---

7. See *Awareness of Dying, op. cit.*

are moved to an intensive care unit, they are quite isolated from people other than the staff, including their families.

All these conditions contribute, without any necessary deliberation by the staff, to the isolation of dying patients. Although a patient may welcome being alone, or alone with kinsmen, he may also fight against his insulation. He may plead successfully to be left with friends and acquaintances, and the staff will wait until he is no longer sentient before moving him. A patient who is already in a single room may devise tactics to get personnel into his room and to increase the time they spend with him, by making urgent demands and complaints or by managing to charm the personnel.

The limits of demand tactics are suggested by what happened to a woman who, like Coleridge's Ancient Mariner, customarily fixed her listeners by the repeated tale of her life. This tactic drove them to countertactics of nonresponse while they busily took care of her creature comforts. A patient can also gain more attention from the personnel if he can charm them. The better they like him, the more contact they are likely to give him anyway, unless his dying distresses them so much that they cannot bear to be around him. As we noted in discussing slow trajectories, a staff member may pull away from a patient not just to minimize contact with him, but to minimize her own emotions and reactions to his story. By avoiding him, she is attempting to lessen the chances of his biography having a lasting impact on her own. On the whole, then, under the kinds of structural conditions noted above it is much easier for patients to gain relative privacy from staff intrusions than to get attention. To the extent that patients fail in either aim, they lose the contest over the shaping of their own trajectories.

We have touched earlier on the staff's occasional efforts to cut down on family visits and banish certain kinsmen from the bedside, as well their attempts to pressure close kin to visit more often. The patient himself may also need to develop tactics to engage or put off his visitors, or to ally his family against the staff or the staff against his family. He complains to family members about his isolation, and gets them to intervene by requesting that they talk with the nurses or protest directly to the responsible physician. With or without prodding, families may attempt to "bribe" the personnel, sometimes successfully, so that their relatives are left less isolated. Or the patient may wish less or more attention from concerned visitors, and accomplishes his aim through negotiation with nurses or physician.

LICENSED BEHAVIOR

Another phenomenon characteristic of the last weeks and days is the license granted patients to engage in otherwise forbidden activities. To the patient previously unaware of oncoming death, this license may help disclose his dying. To the patient already aware, the license may reveal how close his final hours are. However, it may not: for instance, a teenager was allowed to play with a boyfriend on her bed quite out of sympathy for her, but she did not perceive this as license given because she was so near her death. License consists of granting to a patient, sometimes without his requesting it, the opportunity to engage in activities such as eating what he wishes, leaving the hospital to go "for a drive," or going home for the weekend. A nursing student or nursing personnel new to the ward may not recognize that the staff has given up hope for the patient, and may be scandalized at what the patient is allowed to do; the newcomer does not recognize the activity as one "licensed" by certain death. Ulterior motives may be involved in the staff's granting of licensed behavior. By pleasing the patient, they lessen his complaints and make him more tractable and cooperative. Certainly, however, this is not the chief or only motive for granting special dispensations.

As we have noted, a patient sometimes accepts his demise more readily than does the staff. He may press for privileges that the staff is reluctant to grant. The nurses may even warn him that he will hasten his death, but he may not care; he may have devised his own calculus based on a different weighing of values, such as worthwhile living time versus worthless living time. A similar outlook lies behind some patients' refusal to be hospitalized until their final hours, preferring to "live it up" rather than become invalids. Sometimes they hope to die while enjoying themselves, or to die "with their boots on" while working. The patient who knows how to negotiate with the staff, or has various structural conditions working in his favor, can gain more license. Sometimes, however, he may need to obtain it by surreptitious means.

THE PATIENT'S FAREWELLS

Earlier, we touched on the kinsmen's emotionally charged farewells. The patient also may make his farewells. These may not coincide with the leave-taking of his kin; they may not even be visible to his kinsmen. On the other hand, the leave-taking can be mutual and open. Sometimes it is highly ceremonious, as when a European-born American bade his family farewell with a loving, formal speech. He sent them home, said goodbye to his nurses, and died shortly thereafter.

Leave-taking can be terrible for both patient and family, also affecting the interaction between staff and patient. Farewells are especially harrowing when the patient has a while to live but he and his close kin realize how unlikely they are to meet again. Similarly, when the visitors make frequent but not necessarily final farewells, the strain can be quite as great on the patient as on them.

Staff members, too, may suffer both from a patient's poignant farewell, and from their own potential or repeated farewells, whether visible to him or not. A nurse who is much attached to a patient may go off on her weekend or annual vacation uncertain whether the patient will still be in his bed when she returns. While she may prefer *not* to be on duty when he dies, her silent farewell may effectively ruin her time away from the ward. On the other hand, if she dreads his dying when she is away, the leave-taking may be equally difficult for her. Private physicians have also indicated the impact of farewells from patients of whom they are fond.

As we have already pointed out in discussing families, repeated leave-takings can visibly affect the staff's work and collective mood. The effects occur even when a patient has evidenced excellent preparation for his death. The impact is particularly evident when his dying is seen as a considerable social loss. Sometimes when such a patient goes home to die, staff goodbyes are open and poignant.

DECISIVE JUNCTURES

Finally, there are two major critical junctures in the dying trajectory which have immense potential for disturbing either the patient or the work and sentimental orders of a ward. The first occurs when someone decides to prolong the patient's life although others believe he should be allowed to die quickly; the second juncture occurs when someone decides to hasten a patient's death although others believe this intervention should not be made. These decisions sometimes involve the patient's participation—especially the decision to prolong his life, as, for instance, in the choice of an operation that *may* prolong life at the cost of reduced mobility.

The patient's role in the decision not to prolong his dying, or perhaps even to hasten it, is not limited to negotiating with the physician. Patients directly shorten their own lives by various actions—by not eating, or by fatally exposing themselves to cold air at open windows, or, more overtly still, by suicide. Patients who are being kept alive through intravenous feeding or machinery are less likely near the end to kill themselves by pulling out the tubes or by asking that the machinery be turned off; but we have known a successful instance of each of these actions. As we have seen earlier, when patients choose suicide, staff members may be neither unsympathetic nor greatly shocked, providing they can discern an adequate rationale. Unrelenting pain or other physical suffering may seem a sufficient reason for taking one's own life. What would have been upsetting or shocking earlier in the trajectory now is more likely to be condoned. However, the more passive methods by which a patient hastens death are often especially distressing to nursing personnel, for they are cheated of a principal satisfaction in care during the final days: keeping the patient alive and in reasonable comfort and receiving his gratitude for their efforts. Instead the patient is essentially saying—sometimes loudly and clearly—"Go away, there's nothing more you can do for me, let me die."

During most patients' last days, decisions to prolong or shorten life usually are made by the close kin or by physicians, rather than by the patients themselves. Physicians know what patients and families often do not: life can be extended or shortened for at least a few hours or days, and sometimes longer, by various medical tactics. (The ordinary comfort care given by nursing personnel also can extend life, and decisions to reduce that care can reduce the length of a patient's life. By and large, however, nurses and physicians do not seem to think of comfort care alone as requiring deliberate decisions about prolonging or shortening life.)

Several factors bear upon the physician's decision. The nature of the illness is one determinant. During the last days of certain dying patients—for instance, geriatric cases—physicians customarily make no great attempts to stretch out the dying. In general hospitals, however, physicians are more likely to keep life going as long as they judge it sensible to do so; institutional pressures constantly remind them that this is their professional task. Indeed, if a patient unsuccessfully attempts to end his life, physicians are very likely to take drastic steps to prevent renewed attempts. In one instance, at a VA hospital, an elderly patient cut his own throat; a nurse and physician rushed to his rescue, and saved him before they realized that perhaps the rescue made little sense. "Why did we do it?" they asked each other afterward. Another physician remembers a lesson taught him years ago by a patient who literally almost starved himself to death before the physician saved him by forced intravenous feeding. Later the physician was brought up short by the patient's severe questions, asking whether the doctor realized how much will power was involved in deliberate starvation, and did he suppose there was no reason for it?

Like everything else pertaining to slow dying, the decision to prolong or shorten life may need to be made more than once. If kin intervene and beg the physician not to "go all out" for a patient already comatose, or if they are anguished and the physician himself considers a few more days or hours of life senseless, he may take steps not to prolong life. He may cut down on life-prolonging procedures or drugs, may stop blood transfusions, and may even order that some piece of necessary equipment be stopped. Nor is it unknown for a doctor to pass onto a nurse the decision whether or not to prolong life, by signaling that she should or may withhold (or give a bit too much) medication when it seems appropriate.

Nurses in all countries seem to be caught in a structural bind over prolonging or hastening the dying process. By and large, they tend to resist prolongation. They do not always agree with the physician that a patient's life should be prolonged. "What is the sense of it?" they ask among themselves, sometimes even asking the responsible physicians. In American hospitals, nurses frequently show their disagreement openly and may exert direct pressure on physicians. When they do not attempt to influence doctors' decisions, they may harbor disturbing doubts about the paradoxical power of modern medicine, which cannot only sensibly extend life but can also extend it to no good end. We quote from one nurse on a urology ward who unconsciously summed up the dilemma:

If a patient wants to live, then keep giving IV's. This eases it for him and the relative because you are *doing* something. But if he's incurable, why keep him alive? Just ease him out. The difficult stage is not at the very end, anyway. It's before. The period when the patient keeps wanting you to do something more than you're doing. At the end most are unconscious. When they are conscious—saying "save me!"—it's harder—you have to be a stoic not to feel some emotion. It's just as hard when you have one beg you to "let me go!"

She ended her remarks: "I've no answer really."

The probability of nurses' disagreements with physicians increases when a patient consents to becoming a research patient. The physician then is much more open to accusations that he is keeping the patient alive only because of his own research interests. Another condition encouraging disagreements (presumably a rare one, but all the more interesting by contrast) is evident in a situation we encountered in which a nurse, newly graduated from school and also new to the particular ward, found that one of her patients had begun to die. She rushed out and found the resident, but he refused to prolong the patient's life. She was indignant, not knowing the reasoning that lay behind his decision. She believed him simply callous. She did not take into account her own inexperience.

Family members sometimes have a major share in shaping this last phase of the patient's trajectory. Occasionally there may be a conflict between the physician and the family over the family's desire to shorten the ordeal. Thus, one physician brusquely denied the pleas of a mother whose child lay dying inside an oxygen tent. He vowed it was his job to keep patients alive as long as possible. If the patient is dying at home, the family may rush him to the hospital in order to give him a few more weeks or days of life. They may ask the doctor to bring in a consultant, or shop around for another doctor, though usually he cannot prolong the patient's life. In foreign hospitals where family members help with the patient's care, they may help prolong his life through their attentive providing of comfort care. In hospitals in all countries, as we remarked earlier, kin often request the doctor not to prolong the dying. But the doctor in turn may force on them a direct decision as to whether to shorten or prolong life. Rather than precipitate a direct confrontation with the moral decision, the physician may gently ask whether there is "any more we should do," and the relative, sadly or gratefully, or with some other emotion, probably signals "no." Perhaps most often, close relatives either leave the decision up to the doctor, or are unaware that he and the hospital staff explicitly exercise control over shortening or lengthening life.

Which patients, then, are likely to have their lives shortened or prolonged during the last days? We have touched upon most of the structural conditions relevant to that question. The nature of the trajectory, the mode of dying, and the patient's awareness are key variables. Other things being equal, a patient of high social value is likely to elicit staff activity designed to keep him alive longer. The adequacy of hospital and ward equipment has a bearing. Knowledge about this can enhance the patient's or family's power to prolong his life.

The essential issue in these last days is: Who shall have what kinds and degrees of influence in shaping the end of the patient's trajectory? That issue involves not merely how the patient shall die, but also how he shall live while dying. A dying person can hold almost complete control over how he lives his last days by not entering a hospital, or can regain it by leaving the hospital. Lael Wertenbaker's vivid account of her husband's decision to die at home shows how he firmly rejected his doctor's offer of a comfort-giving and life-prolonging operation because of his continued determination to live while dying; as his trajectory departed from his expectations of it, it eventually required rethinking.[8] What is true of patients also is true of doctors, nurses, and families: their decisions also may need to be modified or even reversed during later phases of the trajectory, especially during last days. Insofar as the trajectory takes new directions, new tactics are needed by the agents who try to shape its next phases. However expected may be the physical aspects of a trajectory, the predictions of its psychological aspects—for staff and family as well as for the patient—tend to be less accurate.

Above all, to shape the trajectory during the last days requires juggling tasks, people, and relationships. The legerdemain also requires juggling time: time for tasks, time for people, time

8. *Op. cit.*

for talk. Most subtle of all, the staff is juggling the time still allowed by "fate," since control over aspects of the trajectory may be manageable only for a time, but not forever. These various contingencies are immensely unstable: the patient can be kept unaware just so long; and his family can be kept under control just so long; his family can stand the strain of waiting or of continual farewells just so long; staff can stand for just so long a patient acting unacceptably in the face of death. During the last days, every major person in the dying drama operates within a total context of multiple contingencies. Maintenance of a measure of stability in the ward's temporal order depends on skillful juggling within that context.

IX

Ending the Dying Trajectory

The final stages of dying in hospitals pose three general problems. First, where shall the patient die, at home or in the hospital? Answers to this question may range from a complex decision made by staff, family, and sometimes the patient to a decision by default, which simply leaves the patient wherever he is. Second, the patient's last hours in the hospital require decisions about the kind of career the staff may provide for him as they preside over his death. Specifically, then, in what kinds of work does the staff engage in order to end a dying trajectory appropriately? Third, at this stage of the trajectory the family is usually present and must be managed, with due regard for hospital rules as well as for the death of the patient. How, then, is staff to manage the family, balancing its rights of access and information with the ward's needs, to achieve an atmosphere appropriate to its on-going work?

WHERE TO DIE

Dying in the hospital does not necessarily mean that the patient meets his death in the hospital. He may have spent months dying in the hospital and then die at home, or vice versa. Several conditions and decisions configurate to place a patient in one or the other locale when he reaches the end of his trajectory. The dying patient simply may die where he happens to be if death occurs before a decision can be made or too quickly for one to be made. But in many cases there is time to consider alternatives about where the patient should or could be for his last hours and his death.

No Choice

Various conditions can cause a person to meet death where he happens to be—in the hospital, at home, in the street, and so forth. Most are variants of a single circumstance: sudden dying, the unexpected quick trajectory of a person presumably in good health. However, in the United States, if he is not already in the hospital, and if there is time, the stricken person is usually rushed there. He may die en route, or may get to the ICU or emergency room for a brief dying career.

Sometimes, however, no effort is made to move the patient who starts to die quickly at home. This is most usual when he has been dying for some time. He himself, his family, his doctor and nurses—all may be used to the idea of his dying where he is, and decide, or simply assume, that the process will end there. Even when death is suddenly imminent, they do not feel any urgency to rush him to the hospital, particularly if the chances are slight that he will reach there alive or survive long enough to make a hospital career worthwhile.

In one case, a grandfather, bedridden and ailing for a month at home, felt death approaching and demanded, "Get the women out of the room." They left, interpreting his irritability as due to his illness. When they returned he was dead. Only in retrospect did they realize that he did not want to take any chances on being rushed to the hospital, where they might prolong his life some few days and surely run up a large bill. Thus he managed the end of his own trajectory to—as he saw it—the advantage of his family and according to his wish to die at home.

Sometimes when death is at hand and there is sufficient time for hospitalization, it is nevertheless impossible to move the patient because it might hasten death or because the constant care required during the last hours cannot be interrupted. Then, of course, he dies where he is, irrespective of where anyone wishes him to be. In one case, a lingering patient suddenly started to die quickly of asphyxiation at home in the middle of the night. He could not be moved to the hospital. Since the family were incapable of caring for him adequately, they frantically tried to find a private nurse for his last hours. They could find no one, and so they called the hospital. In an unusual move, the hospital sent a general duty nurse to the home. The nurse ministered to both patient and family. She told us: "It was terrible. The patient had turned black and the family was distraught. This is a good example of why patients should be brought to the hospital to die before it is too late." She felt very strongly that the hospital was the best place to handle the final problems of a dying trajectory, and that a patient should not be left to die elsewhere if it is at all possible to move him to the hospital.

On the other hand, there is sometimes no choice but to have a patient die in the hospital, even if this is unnecessary or even undesirable. The staff may wish to get rid of a patient whose physical death will be easy but whose presence raises excessive social-psychological difficulties on the ward, but sometimes there is no home to which they can send him. Of one such case, a nurse said: "Near the end, after she was supposed to go home and she didn't, she became fairly difficult. She made the staff so uncomfortable they couldn't go near her. But up to then, you know, she was just like most patients."

These instances of patients dying where they happen to be make it clear that this last stage of the dying trajectory is a critical juncture—there are many changes for staff, family, and patient. Medical care changes, and the social and psychological orientations of all parties change. Given these changes, it is not necessarily appropriate for the patient to finish dying where he has been dying. Time permitting, it is frequently desirable for him to be sent home, or to a different ward, or to the hospital.

HOSPITAL OR HOME

The choice of where to end the patient's trajectory hinges on how staff, family, and patient wish it to be managed during the last hours. The choice involves not only physical environment and equipment; it also determines which persons are to preside over the final stage of dying, and the death itself. If the patient is moved, management is, in effect, redelegated. Staff may, for example, redelegate management to the family, possibly providing some equipment or a special nurse. Or the family may delegate management to the hospital.

A patient's earlier dying may have been viewed as a situation calling largely for routine care, whether at home or in the hospital. But the ultimate dying evokes special values and special problems that bear upon how staff, family, and patient consider and relate to each other in deciding where, with whom, and how the patient shall encounter death. Where the person dies becomes the context of what many people consider a special occasion—his death.

Staff. For the staff, the basic issue is whether they have to manage the last hours of the patient's life and, if so, to what degree. The decision typically is made soon after the patient reaches the nothing-more-to-do stage of his trajectory.[1] By then it is fully clear that recovery is no longer a medical possibility. Medical and nursing care now shifts to keeping the patient comfortable until death. Within this context the staff considers where the patient can most conveniently live out his last days, along with the corollary question of who should be in charge of his last hours. Ordinarily, the "who" question for staff is concerned with adequacy of medical or nursing care, not with the patient's social-psychological needs for being with friends or relatives in a certain context at death.

Generally speaking, the staff has several choices as the trajectory moves through the nothing-more-to-do stage up to the last

1. See *Awareness of Dying, op. cit.,* Chapters 11 and 12.

hours. They can send the patient home to die. In most advanced countries, this choice requires a patient whose pain is not overwhelming or uncontrollable, who is not unduly and disturbingly degenerating, and whose last hours will be relatively easy for a nurse or for a family member to handle. Skills and equipment needed at home must be minimal. Any sudden, urgent need for a doctor should be improbable. And, last, the family must want the patient at home.

By and large, staff prefer sending the patient home, as soon as possible after the nothing-more-to-do stage starts. They wish to end his hospital career for several reasons. If possible, they want to spare themselves the ordeal of the last days and hours. They want to release beds for people who can recover—helping patients recover is clearly a preferred challenge. They wish to avoid the family scenes that may occur during the last hours (an attempt to protect the sentimental order of the ward from a special occasion that threatens it).

In some cultures, this preference causes almost routine reaction. In many hospitals in Italy, for example, as soon as there is nothing more to do the family is notified to come and take the patient home. Staff and family agree that it is preferable for the patient to die at home in the "capable" hands of family and priest. It is better that he receive the sacraments there. In the United States, the staff preference is not so readily expressed. Sometimes the staff disregards its own preference and does not ask the family to take him home. In some cases, the family expects a hospital fight to the finish, even if it means some unnecessary prolonging. Or staff may feel that family members are emotionally incapable of taking the patient and supporting his death at home; the hospital is needed to screen them from the ordeal. In these situations, staff sentiments are those expressed by one nurse: "They wish to heaven they could send her home, but they just can't. They don't think the family could tolerate it." When in doubt, they may ask a social worker or public health nurse to check on the family situation to see if it is advisable to ask the family members (or persuade them) to take the patient home, if help from medical personnel, such as a licensed vocational nurse (LVN) or public health nurse, is promised.

The temporal aspect of the decision to send a patient home is variable. The doctor must gauge how much time is left before the end of the trajectory and before it is too late to move the patient. The move may be most appropriate several days or weeks before death, before the hospital becomes the indispensable place to die. Or, if it is necessary to end his trajectory in the hospital, it may still be possible to send him home with the proviso that he return to the hospital when his condition reaches a certain stage before the last hours. Thus the staff spare themselves much of the ordeal of his dying, even if they must minister to his last hours. Returning the patient to a hospital for his last hours may present a problem too. His doctor may be unavailable in time or the ICU full. With little time remaining, a patient may be rushed to a nearby hospital instead of his former hospital. Here the doctors and nurses are strange to a patient and family, who wish to deal with a familiar staff at such a stressful time.

Another temporal aspect of sending a patient home is that while the staff may know that he is going home to die and will not return, the patient or his family may not realize this possibility. The family may think that there is sufficient time to return the patient to the hospital for the last hours, especially if up to this point he had an entry-reentry trajectory. It is typical for the family, and the patient himself, to give the patient more time than the staff does. Indeed, if completely unaware of the patient's condition—as many people in the United States are—the family and patient may think he is going home because he is getting well. And sometimes nobody knows what to think, so they just wait and see.

A third possibility for the staff is to send the patient to a nursing home. This often eases the financial burden and is a frequent resolution to geriatric cases. Or, if money is running out, and the family will not take the patient, or hospital management of the last hours is necessary, then the doctor or administration may put the patient on "research" funds for a few days or send him to a county or state hospital to await death—another frequent solution for geriatric and indigent patients.

In Asia, the staff's desire to get rid of the patient when the doctor gives up hope is partly solved by the "House of Death." Many Chinese feel it is improper to die inside a house of the living. So the family rent a "dying stall" in the House of Death, and call the Sick Receiving Company to transport their sick relative to his cubicle to await death. This house, or block of houses, is financed privately or by the state. Low-caliber nursing is provided. The House handles the problem of old-age dying in the same way as do geriatric wards ("vegetable patches") of our large state hospitals and nursing homes. It provides for the end of the trajectory a career of social death and basic physical sustenance. Patients who can see, live under a condition of constant rehearsal for their own deaths by watching others who are a few days or hours ahead of them. If the family cares to visit or mourn there, a room may be provided or a hallway used, but families do not come frequently.

In many cases, of course, the doctor must decide to keep the patient in the hospital until his death. Because of pain, physical condition, or equipment needs, the patient may not be able to be moved. He may need constant, varying medication that only the hospital staff can administer. His mode of dying may be so distasteful that staff feel it would be unsuitable to force nonprofessionals to put up with the odors, noise, or appearance; in the United States it is the hospital's job to isolate such unpleasantness from family and friends. The patient may have to be watched constantly, or require special equipment. In short, the patient requires care that cannot be provided at home. The staff must see the patient through to the end, even if this care may prolong last days unnecessarily and jar the ward's sentimental order. Many doctors and nurses feel that prolonging a patient's life is not a proper way to end his dying trajectory, but it is hard to stop using the facilities at hand.

Still another possibility when the staff cannot send the patient home is to transfer him to another ward. And indeed, "dumping grounds" develop in the hospital—often an ICU is sacrificed for this purpose. These wards develop characteristics that provide the patient with an appropriate career for ending his trajectory—constant care, watching, and comforts. This career is less readily provided by wards that are designed to handle other stages of the trajectory. For example, a greater number of nurses and immediate access to a resident are usually needed during the last hours, especially if more than one patient is in this stage. Moreover, as we have noted earlier, the sentimental orders of wards handling patients in other stages are usually not well suited to death or an increased rate of death. We see this to some extent in many nurses' eschewal of night duty; they frequently comment that "patients die at night," indicating that putting up with the dying is different than being present at death.

Family. The basic issue confronting the family in deciding where the patient is to die is how they want his last hours to be managed. This issue in turn raises the problem of who should manage these hours to achieve their desires. In considering these two issues, several aspects of the last hours are relevant. "How" includes questions of managing the patient's medical care, of maintaining his physical and psychological comfort, of the possibility of unduly prolonging his life, of the possibility of imposing an excessive burden on the home, of the relative financial costs at home or hospital, and of proper disposal of his body. The problem of "who" will be in charge, either at home or in the hospital, requires consideration of many questions: Will they allow proper ceremonies during the last hours? Will they allow close friends and relatives to be with the patient, or will the patient probably die alone or with unfamiliar people in unfamiliar surroundings? Will the people present at the death bed be able to take the emotional burden? Whether the family actually considers these issues at all (quite aside from whether they consider them "realistically") varies greatly; sometimes there is no time, sometimes the staff alone make and enforce the decisions, or there is no interest.

Prolonging the patient's life is a crucial consideration for family members when deciding where the patient should die. In America, a hospital death means yielding to the staff virtually complete control over his care. The hopsital is equipped for the fight for life, which may impose undue or unnecessary prolonging. But some family members may want every last-ditch effort made. They wish to be able to say to themselves and others that everything that medical science could do was actually done literally "until the very end." Some families feel so strongly about this last effort at prolonging that they send the patient to the hospital even when it is unlikely he will get there alive. In their minds, the "right thing" for the patient is a hospital career at the end of his trajectory.

Some families, however, feel that the sacrifice of a few days or hours of life is a reasonable exchange for the opportunity to die at home. In the following excerpt from "Ezio's Last Days," [2] the wife of Ezio Pinza, the famous singer, tells of making such a decision about her husband.

On May 4th, Dr. Fogel and Dr. Resnik, a renowned consultant, jointly recommended that Ezio be removed to a hospital. Knowing his aversion to hospitals, I asked, "What will be done for him there that cannot be done right here in his own home?" "Nothing in terms of care," the doctors replied. The care I was giving Ezio with the help of Celia and of a wonderful visiting nurse, Miss Lee Vargo, had a quality no hospital could offer. There were, however, several therapies and tests the hospital could give, for which our home was not equipped. "What can this accomplish?" I pressed the doctors, ready to yield at the slightest encouragement. They looked at each other gloomily. At the very best, was the reply, the hospital might save half the man for a brief time. The chances were slim for this as the entire right side was now irrevocably paralyzed. Dr. Fogel mercifully suggested that there was no need to decide immediately. He would be in again later in the day.

2. Epilogue from *Ezio Pinza: An Autobiography* (New York: Rinehart, 1958), p. 278. Robert Magidoff co-authored this autobiography.

Mrs. Pinza had a few hours to decide how and with whom her husband's last hours would be spent. As is typical in such situations, she consulted with a relative and a trusted friend. Both agreed "it would be best to leave Ezio in the peace and dignity of his own home." She almost consulted her oldest child, but felt she was too young for the burden of such a "tragic decision." She then asked her husband, who could not talk but could shake his head; the answer was to stay at home. Mrs. Pinza then called Dr. Fogel and said, "Ezio remains at home." The doctor replied, "I think you have made the right decision. This I say as a friend and as his physician."

Thus the decision to keep the patient at home to die under familiar circumstances was made with the support of several others, including the patient himself. It took into careful consideration the fact that comforting medical care could be supplied as adequately at home as at the hospital. If comfort had been impossible at home, it is likely that the patient would have been sent to the hospital, even if prolonging was also an outcome.

Mrs. Pinza's situation was clear; her husband had only a short time before death. But sometimes the family members must take their option on hospital or home when it is less clear whether the hospital may possibly save the patient. The evidence may indicate that the likely outcome is a useless, costly prolonging, yet family members may not feel convinced and medical personnel in attendance cannot say. "Certainty" is, to be sure, perhaps as much a function of the person as of the evidence. In one such case, a father had a heart attack while hiking in the mountains. The decision fell on the son either to let him die while still pursing his valued way of life or to try to get him to a hospital by helicopter. The chances were that the father would die on the way, or if he arrived alive at the hospital would simply be prolonged a few days. However, one doctor at the hospital could possibly save him with a new procedure. This slight chance was not enough for the son, and he let his father stay, with his wife, in familiar circumstances. He preferred to manage his father's death in a way befitting the way the father had lived, and to leave him in the company of the people whom he loved, rather than providing him a "heroics" career in a hospital. The emotional finesse of such situations is great indeed, for a decision not to send the patient to the hospital for a short prolonging is in effect a decision to let him die.

Once the decision has been made to let the patient die, the family members can exercise control over how he will die. This control is easier to vary and manage in the home than in the hospital because of the greater nonobservability of care given at home. As we pointed out earlier, the hospital staff is in most instances under various pressures to keep the patient alive. Only in infrequent situations of nonobservability do they help him die or provide a set-up for autoeuthanasia. In the home, the family or private duty nurse can easily be more "humane." They can refrain from rescue tactics or can easily discontinue life-sustaining medication or help the patient commit autoeuthanasia. Of course, any such decision is articulated with management of the temporal life of the family and friends present in the home. They cannot be expected to wait days when the patient might be conveniently dead within hours. The question is how best to manage the patient's death amidst these familiar circumstances at home.

Interestingly, whereas families in the United States tend to associate the hospital with prolonging the patient's life, in many sections of Asia and Europe the opposite relationship is seen. Whether justifiably or not, these Asian and European families do not trust the hospital. They often expect the patient's life to be shortened by an unconcerned staff. So they take the moribund patient home to die, telling the hospital staff that if he gets better they will bring him back. This tendency is reinforced by the belief that a person ought to die at home, in familiar circumstances where the right rituals and ceremonies can be performed.

Financial considerations also enter into the family's decision about where to have the patient die. Although private medical insurance and Medicare have in recent years brought about drastic changes in the financial aspects of dying, it is still, for many families, less costly to have their relative die at home. Sometimes they can manage entirely by themselves, or with the help of a night nurse or a day-care "practical nurse." Neighbors may pitch in to help when, say, a mother must shop or work, but this generosity lasts only so long, and can easily run out before the constant watch maintained during the last hours. On the other hand, if the patient can die in a state or county hospital as a free patient, or on a health insurance plan, the family may find it financially advantageous to send him to the hospital for his last days, so that they do not have to hire home nursing care.

In various countries, cultural factors influence the cost considerations. In *one Italian city,* for example, death away from home raises a unique cost problem. It costs more to ship a body home in a hearse for burial than to send a live person home in a cab. Thus, the location of the patient during his last hours can be critical for poor Italian families. The question of cost adds to their wish to get him home for the end of his trajectory. If they cannot move him or if there is no time, the family may conspire with the hospital nuns to send the body home as if the patient were alive. They even postpone the sacraments in order to add to the pretense. The sentimental order of these hospitals supports such a move (a false end to the trajectory), even if the sacraments are given late. Indeed, if a physician signs a death certificate before the body has been moved home, the rest of the staff may become furious with his lack of concern for the family's budget.

In considering the problems of prolonging and finances, family members must take into account the burden of care that will fall on them if the patient spends his last hours at home. We have mentioned the problems of whether they can provide the necessary physical care and whether they can endure the death emotionally. Another problem is whether they have suitable space at home for him. Although the patient may have shared a room while in good health, usually it is preferable that he be segregated from the family while dying. If segregation is not practicable— as in small urban apartments or small houses—it may be too much of a burden to keep the patient at home during his last hours. His presence would be too pervasive, would dominate too much the lives that must go on while he dies. The space problem is especially difficult for the poor who live in cramped urban settings.

Other aspects that the families consider are how "humanely" they want the patient treated and what kinds of company and ceremonies they want for him. Americans, as we have said, by and large take it for granted that the hospital is the place to die; it is equipped to handle the medical burden of the last hours. It is mainly hospital staff members who wish the patient to die at home, if possible. But Americans also want hospital death to be "humane." Families express this wish in the common preference for retaining more social-psychological control over the patient's last hours, leaving to the staff the management of medical and nursing care. Family members want as much chance as possible to be with him, and want staff members to be more considerate of the social-psychological dimensions of staff relationships (such as talk, attention, and information) with the patient during his last hours. The family wants to be present during the last hours, be continually informed, hold the patient's hand, and talk with him.

In many hospital situations, however, kinsmen are put in a waiting room and are forbidden to be with their loved one at the end. They are told that their presence is too stressful for the patient, who "must rest" as he dies. But they are not told that their presence is likely to threaten the sentimental order of the ward, and so disrupt work. It might disturb the staff to see the family mourning with the patient; it might disturb other patients to witness scenes of what is possibly in store for them. If the family loses composure in public during these intense hours, then surely everyone will be upset. The staff's solution, most generally, is to let family members visit for short periods and remain in the waiting room as long as they like, but to suggest they go home for rest. Thus the probability is low that kinsmen will be with the patient at death, even if they are waiting just down the hall from him. Consequently, they will experience his death as an announcement, not a graceful passing.

In sum, Americans tend to accept the patient's death in the impersonal hospital, where "the ebb and flow of events is controlled by routine and by strangers," instead of at home, in familiar circumstances and among familiar people. Yet at the same time they wish more control over whom he is with and how his last hours with these people are socially managed. Kinsmen wish to make certain he dies with familiar company, if not surroundings not with strangers or alone, as is liable to happen in the hospital.

In Europe and Asia, as we have noted, families generally feel that the patient ought to die at home in familiar circumstances, in his own bed. So they accept, if they can manage the situation, the doctors' sending him home—or they just take him home. One reason for this stand is their wish to engage in ceremonies in conjunction with the patient's passing. Ceremonies—both religious and familial—have an important role in America, too, but they are arranged rather differently.

The family gathering at the patient's bedside is easier to handle at home, although there is always the problem of timing the gathering of kin with the death. However, at home the family can wait while doing other things, can easily gather periodically to chat with the patient, and can rush to his bedside when his time comes. This kind of gathering is especially appropriate for an aged parent or grandparent, but can occur for all family members, young and old. It is considered desirable in Asia, but in the United States tends to be overlooked or neglected in favor of having a few intimates next to the patient while he receives medical and nursing care in the hospital. At home, the family gathering can continue as a wake for the patient, which Asians prefer. In America, the family must go to the funeral parlor several hours after the death. As one family member said after a hospital death, "They won't even leave the poor body around long enough for a wake." In Asian and some European hospitals, there is likely to be a chapel or funeral room in which the family continue their gathering as a wake.

Provision for religious ceremonies is more or less standardized in American hospitals. As a patient nears death, some have a routine procedure for calling a chaplain of the correct faith. The problem for the staff is timing, for they may call the chaplain too late or too soon; either error upsets the family and patient. Staff also must be able to reach the chaplain in time. If the priest whom they usually call is unavailable, then they must find another one somewhere, and fast. Also, they are sometimes not certain of the religion of the patient if it is not marked on his record, or may not know if the patient or family wishes a particular form of last rites. The family may not be at hand, or the patient may be comatose. In the emergency ward, it is fairly often impossible to figure out what to do about a religious ceremony.

All in all, the American family in abdicating control to the hospital over the last hours does so knowing that the staff will arrange for religious ceremonies if necessary. In Asia and some European countries, the family will arrange for them in the hospital but prefers to have them at home, linked with the family gathering. The home is where ceremonies can be done "properly," to the comfort of the family as well as the patient.

Sometimes in the American hospital the sacraments are given to a sentient patient who did not know he was dying and whose family is not present. "This situation is enough to scare a patient to death," a chaplain in such a case told us. He was also distressed for another reason: "The thing that shook me is that she died so quickly, and I had more to say to her." Mistiming in the family's calling for the chaplain is more likely in the hospital than at home because they may not immediately learn of, or be able to observe, changes in the patient's condition. In the home, it is more feasible to alert the clergyman in advance and then have him call back frequently to inquire when he will be needed, thus forestalling delays and mistiming. He can then come in time to comfort the family and perform last rites. But this repeated calling is bothersome to staff in the hospital, and they are not too likely to give adequate information until they are ready to call the chaplain.

The family can make or participate in the decision of where the patient is to die only if they have the time and are given or take the opportunity to do so. Then they balance out the several factors we have discussed. While individual cases vary, the national patterns are clear enough. In the United States, it is increasingly unusual to have a patient at home for his death, but in Asia and in some European countries it is unusual to leave a patient in the hospital for his death.

The Patient. For the patient, the basic issue about where to die is how he wishes it managed and with whom he wants to be. During the last hours many patients have no choice—they are dying too quickly, are comatose or not lucid enough to decide, or require hospital care that cannot be given at home. Some patients have no home or their kinsmen cannot take them. Some are not aware they are dying, and thus are denied a choice, even though they would prefer to die at home.

Several factors are typically involved in a patient's own decision to remain in the hospital. Even if he can leave the hospital, he may wish to stay because he expects the pain during the last hours to be great, and feels more sure of having a painless death in the hands of skilled staff members rather than a distressed family and a single nurse. Or the patient unable to take care of himself may wish to stay in the hospital so as not to be a burden on his family. Geriatric patients, particularly, feel that their care would be too burdensome for their aged spouses, children, or grandchildren. These elderly persons often have acute insight about the situation. Sometimes an aged parent believes that his effect upon the people with whom he lives is destructive. These geriatric patients choose nursing homes or hospitals as locales in which to end their trajectories; frequently this choice is also an acknowledgment of their low social loss to family life. (One highly emotional housewife in her 40's exclaimed that she would never be able to live in her house again if her aged father were to die there.) In contrast, younger adults who are dying worry less about their possible burden on wives and parents, for they sense that their social loss to family life is high, and that the family therefore will be more tolerant of the burden.

Fear of rejection by the persons the patient wants to have with him at death may also keep him from leaving the hospital.

He may realize that a person about to die does not make very pleasant company, that the very imminence of death, as well as an intolerable or repugnant physical condition, may repulse even his intimate family. This fear distresses the dying patient, especially since his self-confidence is likely to be low; he may therefore prefer the impersonal isolation of the hospital staff to the risk of being isolated by the family he loves. Thus, an American patient, when wishing to go home to die among familiar circumstances and companions, thinks twice about what he has to offer, for his trajectory at this stage may well be unacceptable to others at home. In America, he knows, dying persons are typically avoided even by kinsmen. Dying among family at home becomes only a valued abstraction. So he chooses to die on a ward where his trajectory is acceptable and where he is sheltered from possible rebuffs by his family. In Europe and Asia, the home is still a more acceptable context for death.

If conditions do permit his dying at home—his condition is not too repugnant; the family wants him, will not avoid him, and will take the burden; his pain can be managed sufficiently well— the patient is likely to ask to die there. He will prefer this because dying at home gives him a greater chance to manage his own trajectory. If he gives orders to the hired nurse and family members caring for him, there is a greater probability that they will grant his wishes than that the hospital staff would. He is not in competition with other patients. He has a greater chance to control and negotiate his medicine and care in order to relieve pain more completely or to reduce prolonging. One patient kept asking to leave the hospital. Since she continually needed suctioning, the staff suspected that she wanted to die within hours at home—she was, in fact, trying to manage the end of her trajectory.

During the last hours of constant care, the patient is often especially sensitive about getting various attentions from the people around him. Hence, as he moves into this stage of his trajectory, it is particularly attractive to the patient to be at home, where he is not in competition with other patients. By contrast, during last hours in the hospital he must be screened off from other patients in order not to provide them with a disturbing death rehearsal. At home he is spared this isolation from friendly patients, which is enforced by hospital rules, yet he is provided with privacy.

In wishing to die at home, the patient typically focuses strongly on the companionship of the closest family member— parent, spouse, or child. In the stress of the last days and hours, he may not wish to see other kin or friends except for brief moments, but may desire the one intimate family member to be present constantly. The burden on this one member is much greater than on the other relatives or friends; he may be virtually trapped at the bedside until the patient's death. Amazingly enough, the dying patient often recognizes that the home setting is better able than the hospital both to permit this entrapment and to make it tolerable for his dear one.

In one case, an aging husband, all functions gone and inching toward death, wanted only his wife with him and no one else— no family, friends, or nurse. She ministered to his condition constantly and dared not leave him for more than fifteen minutes. The rest of the family wondered how she could endure it. The patient during his last hours was in no condition to worry about the burden he put on her; and the wife "stuck it out." In this way, when a hospital career is traded for a home career, the last days and hours may irreversibly trap a strong, intimate family member into managing the end of the trajectory. The entrapment can end only if the patient loses consciousness or dies quickly, or if the family member breaks down.

LAST HOURS IN THE HOSPITAL

The patient's hospital career changes as he enters the last hours of his trajectory. As we have noted, this stage usually requires several changes in medical and nursing care. In earlier chapters, we have already mentioned some of the special features of care during quick dying, in which the last hours or minutes are sometimes filled with medical heroics. Here we shall discuss the more general aspects of hospital care that come into play as the patient is about to die. Three discernible stages arise during the last hours of the trajectory: the death watch, the death scene, and the death itself.

THE DEATH WATCH

The death watch is "empty" time. It is the lull before the storm. It is the time before the potential crisis scene starts, when nothing is happening to the patient. Since the death watch is an empty temporal space, and since the staff always have much to do, there is a great temptation to neglect it. For several significant reasons, however, someone, preferably a staff member, must watch the patient constantly.

The most important of these reasons is the patient's anticipated physical condition, upon which hinge the work and sentiments required to start the ending of the patient's trajectory at the right moment. He must be watched constantly so that split-second constant care can be given immediately when necessary, to prevent, if possible, the dying scene; for example, preventing him from choking to death by holding him upside down, giving medication every ten minutes, keeping him bundled or cool, or keeping him suctioned. Quite often nurses feel very strongly that nothing should be left undone that might prevent the dying scene, so they are intensely involved in the death watch and do everything possible up to the very last minute. This forestalls any feeling of negligence, even if the significance of their care is ambiguous. For example, keeping the patient free of pain can be a particularly difficult task at the end; if the patient cannot talk and is immobilized, or has high tolerance to pain killers, success may be highly debatable.

The death watch is also required for physical control of the patient when the end starts. The patient often is asleep or comatose during the watch, and then, when the crisis of dying starts, he sometimes wakes and becomes violent or at least hyperactive. He may toss and turn and displace tubes or hit equipment alongside his bed. He may even hurt others. We were told by a navy corpsman, experienced at death watches, that sailors tend to react to their last war scene when they wake up. In one case, he had to hold a patient down while ringing for help.

Verbal control may also be needed. A patient at the brink of death sometimes becomes, in a way, mentally ill, and feels a license to say what he pleases. He may swear, insult, accuse, or reveal information that should not be heard by family members waiting at the deathbed; and must then be calmed, tranquilized, screened, or separated from his family. Such verbal deviances can easily shake up the ward's sentimental order, which at this point of impending death may be quite vulnerable.

A very important aspect of the death watch is its role in maintaining the sentimental order of the staff members, by assuring that the patient will not die alone. This consequence, a by-product of the attention given the patient, may not be talked about or formally recognized, but it is strongly felt among many staff members whether they are aides, nurses, or doctors. Its importance is revealed, in part, when there is no death watch. When medical or nursing care does not require a watch, nurses can be heard voicing dismay over the patient's being alone. One student said she "couldn't believe the patient would be left alone." Part of the concern arises because leaving the patient to die alone may provide a demoralizing death rehearsal to other patients if they observe that patients can die alone in this hospital. Indeed, since staff members and family members will also die sometime, they may also feel demoralized about a death rehearsal which has no death watch.

The death watch also serves as a way of handling family members who wish to be at the deathbed at the right time. Their awareness that the staff is watching and will notify them when to come to the hospital, or bring them in from the waiting room, keeps them quiet and waiting until the death scene. The staff can say, "Go home and get some rest, we'll call you." If it is not appropriate for family to participate in the death scene, the death watch is a way of keeping them waiting at a distance until they are told of death. To be sure, the death watch may not indicate an accurate timing of the death, and then the staff may not reach the family in time for their arrival to the bedside. Or the death may occur at night, and the night staff may not have time to call the family or may not be aware that the family is waiting at home. Sometimes it is suitable for a strong family member to serve in the death watch. He may not be aware of this; he is just told that he can remain as long as he wants and "please call the nurse if a sudden change occurs" in the patient. All in all, whatever the details, the death watch, by providing continual information on the patient, provides a lever for controlling the family either by giving the family member a legitimate place in, or by keeping him out of, the last hours of the patient's trajectory.

Several differentials in awareness of dying and in the temporal whereabouts of people may prevent the death watch. A patient who is awake and aware of impending death may not wish a death watch. He may request to be alone, though often patients ask for someone to be with them. On the other hand, the patient's unawareness may prompt the staff not to watch because it does not wish to scare him about his fate. "What is this, a death watch?" demanded one patient, asking everyone to leave the room; the staff then had to engage in surreptitious, intermittent watching. Sometimes a patient announces that he is dying, but the staff members do not think so. If he is correct, he dies alone, with no farewells to family members. Such a death shatters the sentimental order of the ward. In one case, a head nurse, anticipating this possibility, complied when a patient asked to have his wife called. The wife came and he died; the nurses were relieved that they had complied.

Often there is no death watch until the doctor says the patient is in his last hours. If the doctor is not near at the right time and cannot be reached readily, the nurses take it upon themselves to start the watch, based upon their own knowledge or symptoms the doctor has told them to watch for. Thus the existence of awareness about certainty and time of death, and the degree of credibility others put in the awareness are crucial conditions for starting the death watch.

On the other hand, sometimes a watch is started but the patient does not die—he only goes through a rehearsal for what he will go through if he does die. And there may be more than one false watch. If they happen too often, these watches can be very disturbing to staff and family, especially as they may find themselves beginning to wish that the patient would die.

Instituting a death watch often creates a personnel problem, even on quick-dying wards that have more nurses than the medical wards. No ward is geared to provide enough staff for a constant watch by trained personnel. In short, on all wards the death watch is somewhat of a disrupting, unacceptable aspect of the trajectory, although something must be done to provide for its occurrence. Therefore hospitals and staff have developed several strategies to handle this invasion of the "normal" workload, which soaks up valuable nursing time despite little gain. A hospital may simply require the regular ward staff to handle the problem on their own. But the hospital may provide measures—some of which we have already mentioned—to ease the impact on the work order.[3]

A hospital can hire special aides as "sitters." A denominational hospital may use a religious hospital volunteer (e.g., a retired nun). A navy corpsman told us that his unit treated the death watch as an extra-duty assignment, much like KP or guard duty. Hence the work and sentimental order was not disturbed, since extra duty work is required of all corpsman a few times a month. A hospital can also provide or let develop a "dumping ground," such as a special ICU, with enough personnel to preside simultaneously over several death watches. Another strategy is to relax visiting rules so that family members can serve as helpers

3. One solution is to require no death watch—to avoid the problem entirely. This approach we found in a chronic TB hospital in Scotland. The nature of the disease and the long duration of hospitalization make pinpointing the death watch extremely hard. Patients usually linger in the same state for months, then suddenly die.

day and night. Or the hospital may just ignore the work shift problem posed by a death watch. That is, a ward that can handle the watch during the day and evening shift may be too under-staffed to manage during the night shift. If death does occur at night, staff on the day shift who have worked hard with the patient "become [as one nurse said] very upset about the fact that he died without close observation." Questions arise, but little is done about the nonobservance of death watches.

The staff have their own strategies, which vary considerably by ward. On the ICU, the doctor himself may watch for several hours while waiting for a chance to save the patient. Sometimes patients who may still have a chance are sent to the ICU for this type of watch. But doctors with patients on other wards may watch if the case is very complex, sufficiently interesting, or personally involving. And hospital doctors (especially residents) have more opportunities to engage in death watches, or at least to keep constant tabs on patients, than private doctors who have many demands calling them outside the hospital.

Without the doctor present, the nursing staff develops several tactics for handling the watch without letting it interrupt adequate care for the other patients. Nurses may get an alert, recovering patient to watch; patients frequently like to be helpful if they are up to the task. Sometimes they do not know that they are handling a death watch; they simply report a change in condition. And the nurses themselves develop variations of teamwork for the watch. For example, they leave the door open so that every nurse "pops in" for a quick look as she goes by. This tactic gives fairly good coverage. Nurses take turns sitting at the bedside or, if they have a patient or family member watching, may take turns answering calls to the room. They may also take turns covering a nurse's other duties when she is busy with a death watch, relieving her for meals, comforts, and emotional strain. Nurses also use ward clerks or aides for the death watch, or to cover for a nurse who must temporarily abandon the watch. In short, no matter who is on watch, the variation in teamwork provides "backstoppers" who relieve and check with the watcher. This arrangement also reduces the loneliness of the watcher, who is doing nothing active most of the time while alone with the dying patient. Thus, backstopping is important in preserving the sentimental and work orders of the wards.

Handling the death watch may also have a spatial aspect. The staff may reserve a room or space near the nursing station in which the patient can be watched easily. If more than one patient requires constant watching, they can be placed in the same area and watched by one nurse.

THE DEATH SCENE

The death watch terminates with the patient's actual moments of "passing." At this point, the watcher calls the doctor and other nurses to help the patient die comfortably. This portion of the trajectory is very short, but in the few cases observed and reported several problems emerged.

Nurses prefer *not* to be present at death. They prefer to avoid the potentially awful "last look" of the patient, as well as other unpleasant aspects of the end of dying. One nurse put it as simply, "The worst part of nursing is having to watch someone die." Another said, "He looked badly—just at the last moment." Several nurses have told how the patient "turns black." Others report how "his eyes and mouth were open." A student nurse, in anticipation of being present at her first death scene, was already preparing to control herself for the event: "I don't know what my reaction will be when I see my first death. My instructor suggested that the first time we note what is happening physically, or leave the room if you can't take it, try and learn to control yourself, emotions are awfully important, that you could get something out of it then." Nurses find the death scene upsetting; the threat to the sentimental order of the ward increases with the number of deaths and the number of nurses who must witness them.

The sentimental order can also be jarred by being present at death when the patient "doesn't look like he is dead." This can be "disappointing" to nursing personnel, as one nurse explained.

The continuing look of life makes the death more poignant. It reminds viewers more of the life that was, whereas looking dead finalizes death. Moreover, the patients who are most likely to look alive at death are the younger adults and children, whose social loss is great.

Because of their aversion to being present at death, nurses develop and employ several strategies for avoiding this phase of the dying trajectory. These strategies are, for the most part, worked into the on-going career that is provided the patient in his last hours. They depend on the probabilities of being elsewhere, which derive from the structural conditions and schedules of work and from the short span of the death scene. The probability that a nurse will be present at death is higher than for a doctor or an aide; but the probability for any particular nurse is, of course, low. So the individual nurse focuses on the structural probability that she will not be the nurse who is there, and tries to increase it.

For example, she is on duty only one-third of the day; she believes, not without foundation, that patients tend to die at night, and so tends to avoid the night shift on wards where many patients die. But even if she is on the night shift, the nurse tries to choose conditions under which, if on a death watch, she may conveniently and "accidentally" be away through the death as the patient sleeps through it. She tries to choose wards where not many patients die. When a patient's death is near, she takes a few days of weekend vacation time or gets sick. She gets assigned to a short trajectory ward where, although many deaths occur, the doctor is often with the patient as he dies. The nurse immerses herself in the hustle and bustle of the ward, leaving the doctor himself at the death scene. She uses the staff rotation system to avoid a death, juggling her transfers between wards or refusing transfers to wards where many die. A nurse may also use other patients' claims for attention in order to avoid a death scene; she asks another nurse or an aide to cover for her during the twenty minutes that she is away from the bedside. Nurses can also request a different set of patients to care for on the same ward. Sometimes this is done with clear purpose, a nurse "trading off" a dying patient for another or "pleading off" the case with the head nurse, because during the death watch she realizes, "If I stay in there any longer, I'm going to crack, so something has got to be done." Sometimes this occurs through the normal switching of patients for a nurse on the ward.

The nurse may time her departure for other duties to coincide with letting a family member watch for a while at the bedside— then it may be too late for her to be called before the death. This raises the question of under what conditions staff may allow family members to witness the death scene. One major condition is that the patient be dying comfortably and acceptably; that is, he is neither in great pain nor in a physical state or aspect of care that would unduly distress the family. Preferably, the staff should also have reason to believe the family member will be able to confront the death with composure. In the course of the patient's trajectory, family members develop reputations as to their abilities to control themselves. The relative with no known reputation or with a poor one is unlikely to be permitted at the death scene, for the staff wishes to avoid emotional outbursts that disturb the patient, other patients, and themselves. If a kinsman has a poor reputation, he will simply not be called in time. If the family becomes angry, they are told that no one knew when the trajectory would end.

If the relative has a good reputation, every effort may be made to have him at the death. He still may miss it because of maltiming or surprises. In one case, "the wife went home for half an hour to wash and change clothes," and missed her husband's death, which she would have been permitted to attend. She had been sitting with her husband for two weeks and had developed among the staff a reputation for composure and preparation. In fact, the nurses were distressed that she had missed the death. Sometimes the family member is not at the hospital, but the death can be postponed several hours until he arrives from work or home. In one instance, death was postponed a day while a son returned from New York to his father's bedside in Los Angeles.

Ethnic background also influences staff views about kinsmen. As we have noted in the United States as well as in their native countries, Italians and Greeks tend to be considered as very expressive and it is feared they will create scenes. Scots and English are considered stoic and to be depended upon for composure even though they may be breaking down inside. By and large, the Anglo-Saxon attitude is considered desirable for Americans. In any event, the American hospital tolerates only a scene of minor proportions at death. Staff members are prepared to help the members through it. Doctors murmur assurances, nurses console; chaplains, social workers, and sisters may be made available by the hospital to rescue the kinsmen from the death scene itself.

X

After Death in the Hospital

The patient's trajectory ends with his death. But the hospital's work is not finished. It must dispose of the body; it must wind up its relationship with the family; it must write a conclusion to the patient's story. Hospitals are well organized for disposing of the body, but they vary in procedures for disposing of the family and have little or no organization for ending the patient's story—the staff does this latter task on its own, as any particular story seems to require. It is generally felt that the sooner the hospital achieves these dispositions the better, so pressure is put on the staff to expedite them.

The three dispositions are highly interrelated. The tenor and circumstances of how the family is handled determine in large measure how and when the body is removed to the hospital morgue and funeral home, as well as how the patient's story is brought to a close. There is, nevertheless, much independent variation among disposition careers provided for these "remains." We shall consider first the family, then the body, and finally the patient's story.

DISPOSING OF THE FAMILY

"Disposing of" the family is a situational requirement for hospitals and their staffs. If, at the time of death, the family is at home, there is usually no time or need for them to come to the hospital. The doctor or a staff member notifies them by phone, and they next see the body of their kinsman at a designated funeral home. But when the family members are on the premises the hospital must deal with them. This task has many ramifications.

THE DEATH ANNOUNCEMENT

If family members are at the hospital but not at the death scene, the death first must be announced to them. Several conditions give this crucial announcement greater or less potential for creating a "wailing scene" that may disturb the ward. Various conditions of the patient's dying trajectory, as well as the kinsmen's reputation for behavior, which has developed among staff, will have provided some indication of how they will react to this announcement.

If, during a lingering trajectory, the family have been made aware by successive preannouncements that the patient was dying, and have also been told when he was likely to die, then staff usually expect them—or at least the strongest member—to be able to take the news with composure. Little explanation is required. Nor is any special announcement ritual needed. Almost any of the nurses or residents can convey the news; it can be passed on in the hallway, or waiting room, or even at the nursing station. Under this configuration of conditions, the death announcement is, in effect, the confirmation of a long-expected event. Since this is the easiest interactional situation for staff to handle at this trying moment, some doctors and nurses try whenever possible to prepare family members by keeping them continually informed. Once told of the dying trajectory, some family members, too, try to create a reputation for being easily informed, so as to encourage staff unhesitatingly to make successive preannouncements and the death announcements on time.

It is more difficult to announce death when the family of the lingering patient has been "left out" of the dying situation—when they have not been made clearly aware of the approach of death. They may have been denied access to clues or may have perceived them ambiguously; or they may have pretended not to recognize them. In any case, if kinsmen's knowledge of impending death has not been clear or has been denied in the eyes of staff, their reputation is one of less than adequate preparation, indicating that they are likely not to take a simple death announcement well. The news must then come from the doctor, the only legitimate source of such information; some sort of explanation is needed to fill in their vague knowledge and erase their doubts or denial of what had been happening earlier. The explanation usually includes a temporalized resumé of the dying trajectory and the hospital career provided for it: "As you know, his chances weren't very good, but we did everything we could." If possible, the announcement is made in an office or an empty room in order both to provide a quiet, somewhat formal setting for the solemn news and to insulate family reactions. These crucial announcements, then, are spatially and temporally managed with care to avoid scenes that may spill over to disrupt the sentimental order of the ward.

Announcing death to family members of a patient whose death ended a quick dying trajectory is usually difficult. There has been little time to prepare them. Preannouncements a few days ahead are few, brief, and usually grave. The death itself must be announced while family members are still trying to accept the fact that the patient is dying. However, explanations of quick death are generally specific, and the death announcement ("He had a coronary") may not require any addition to what the preannouncements provided. Therefore, the announcement can be made by a nurse as well as the doctor. The fact of death is all that needs to be communicated, and the intensity of care at the death might prevent the doctor from appearing as speedily as the nurse. But with the announcement must come consolations about the rapidity of the dying trajectory. The nurse expects to spend some time in helping the family remain composed; if her consoling is not adequate, she may call other nurses, aides, chaplains, nuns, clerks, or other family members, depending on who is available for such backstopping. The doctor may be called upon later to provide explanations as to why medical science cannot as yet prevent this kind of quick death. In all these cases, too, an effort is made to provide privacy for the announcement.

As we saw in Chapter VII, the unexpected quick death comes as a surprise to the family. With no preannouncement to help prepare the family, staff have no idea how they may react. They usually expect the worst. Moreover, since the unexpected quick death is also a surprise to staff members, they must, first of all, announce the death to each other and maintain or regain their own composure. Then one of them—preferably the doctor, who can legitimize the death and its suddenness—approaches the family, usually ushers them into the privacy of a closed room, and engages in a "prolonged announcement." That is, he builds up to the news of the death. This build-up describes the patient's condition, tells what he was doing before the surprise, and explains why saving him was impossible. Then follows a more general explanation about how people die this way, why death cannot be forestalled by medicine, or under what conditions it could be prevented. This general kind of announcement may be truncated by a doctor who is too upset to go on. Or the announcement may be stopped also by family members going into shock, wailing loudly, threatening suicide, or making accusations. Further talk is not meaningful.

Without any reputation for potential behavior, kinsmen are fully expected to "go to pieces" until they prove otherwise to staff. Doctors and nurses have several coping strategies in this explosive situation. Personnel on emergency wards are especially adept at these strategies. For example, if an accident case is brought in DOA ("dead on arrival") or dies soon after entry, his family may initially be notified that he has had an accident and that his condition is undetermined but could be grave. Or on a medical ward the nurse phones and says, "The patient has taken a turn for the worse. Would you please come?" Thus the trip to the hospital gives family members time to get somewhat used to the idea of possible death, even if they can hardly be expected to be adequately prepared for it. The nursing staff also likes such strategies because they feel the doctor should be the one to announce the death.

A similar false preannouncement leading to brief preparations may be used for families who are at the hospital waiting for news about someone in the ICU, in surgery, or in the emergency ward, when the timing of the death allows the staff a chance to act as if the dying trajectory were still in progress. The staff can then, since the family cannot invade the sick room or get information elsewhere, have time to wait before giving the death announcement. This situation may be created even if the family is at the patient's bedside when he suddenly starts to die quickly. The alert nurse quickly ushers the family out, saying that the patient requires a quick treatment or procedure done in private. The mildly panicked family then waits until the nurse reports on the patient, preparing themselves for the worst. The nurse must find a doctor both to pronounce death and then to tell the family. If none is immediately available, and if she fears the family may come back into the patient's room to see what is going on, she may then announce the death herself. This alternative of earlier announcing outside the room reduces the dangers of a potential scene.

Another strategy is to choose the best person for giving the surprise announcement, letting the doctor explain later. The person may be someone who is good at giving consolation, such as a social worker, a chaplain, or a nun. Or it may be someone close to the family—a friend who has visited with them, or, after an accident, the family doctor who has been called. The family may be sized up quickly and then the strongest member told, leaving to him the job of telling others in the family. These strategies build into the announcement a variety of specialized people who are ready to help the family through the shock and to prevent scenes. In any case, the staff stands ready to tranquilize or sedate and possibly provide a hospital bed to any family member needing it.

The importance both of preparation and of careful strategy in announcing a death is highlighted by instances in which neither was used. In one unusual case a physician on an emergency ward, shocked at the death of a patient, ran to the waiting room and told the mother, who suspected nothing, that her son had just died. The woman shrieked and wailed. Others in the waiting room became highly agitated. The nurses, horrified at what the doctor had done, attempted to restore calm to the doctor as well as to the visitors. When the doctor recovered, he returned to the grieving woman and with apologies took her into a private office and started to explain what he knew of the sudden death— an effort that also consoled the staff.

Sometimes, regardless of the preannouncement conditions or the kind of death, a doctor who finds this job particularly difficult finds ways to avoid announcing to the family. He may leave the hospital before the death, giving no instructions but knowing that in his absence someone else must announce to the waiting family. Or, upon leaving, he may instruct the nurse to tell the family members (whom he had told the patient was dying) if the patient should die. One nurse caught in this situation realized that the doctor had slipped away precisely to avoid the death announcement. She became furious. Her countertactic was to notify the doctor and "let him tell the family." A doctor might answer with an "order" for the nurse to call the family. Other nurses have suffered through their anger or have turned the task over to the resident who pronounced the death. Doctors tend to use this tactic to avoid being bothered at night.

Successive preannouncements do not necessarily prepare family members adequately. Indeed, their preannouncement reactions may establish for them poor reputations for maintaining composure. They cry too easily and too loudly, faint or become accusing, barrage staff with questions without listening to the answers, or ask unanswerable questions ("Why him of all people?") Announcements are made to such family members as carefully as to the unprepared kinsmen during a quick, sudden trajectory. Again, the strongest member may be told, and sent home with the family with orders to tell them there. In some cases, staff almost never directly inform certain family members, either for the time being or "forever"—for example, relatives who are severely ill themselves, mothers of premature babies, or aged grandparents who might die from the news. The hospital then may search for a strong family member to tell—usually a distant relative—asking him to sign necessary papers. A husband of a wife who has given birth to a "preemie" who then dies may receive an immediate announcement and be asked to tell his wife when she wakes or is "ready" for the news.

THE LAST LOOK

There are several distinct phases of the end of the trajectory when family members may take their last looks at the patient. They may do so during a farewell or during the death watch; at death, if they participate in the death scene; or after death in the hospital, before his body is sent to the funeral home. Some do not take a last look, preferring to remember the patient "as he was."

The hospital staff is usually generous in allowing the last looks before death. Indeed, sometimes they suggest them. "Now you go over and look at him tonight," said one nurse to a mother, implying that she might never see him alive again. After death, however, staff seldom suggest a last look. It is unusual to hear a nurse say after death, as one did, "You can see the patient if you wish." For staff members consider the risks of emotional upset during an after-death last look too great, particularly if the mode of death is not "viewable" to laymen. Moreover, it is an unusual hospital indeed which has personnel both available and prepared for the task of ushering the family into the room for its look and handling the consequences for the sentimental order.

Requests for such post-death last looks mainly occur on the quick-dying wards (ICU, operating room, emergency, and premature babies). On these wards family members usually are not allowed at the death scene, since their presence would interfere with the intense efforts to save the patient. As we have stated, these families are relatively unprepared for the death. They may not have had any chance to see the patient after the quick trajectory started, and hence are not directly aware of his often drastically changed appearance. Yet, precisely because they have not seen the patient during his dying, they are likely to need a last look after death, to say goodbye and to recognize the reality of the death. They wish to see for themselves; they wish to come to terms with the *mystic gap* between their kinsman alive and their kinsman suddenly and astoundingly dead. Hence, after announcing death the doctor must be ready to manage the family's request for one last look at the patient.

On the lingering dying wards, requests for a last look after death are less frequent, and those who ask are likely to be better able to maintain composure. Family members, unless kept completely unaware, usually have had sufficient time to make farewells and take tentative last looks before death, and to become prepared for the death. As we have pointed out, intimate family members often participate in the death scene and thus have a last look at the time of death.

When relatives request or even demand a last look at the body before it goes to the funeral home, the doctor or nurse's decision rests on several conditions. First and foremost, the possibility of a scene (especially in cases of quick deaths) is considered. How insistent is the family member? Insistence itself is prime evidence for the probability of a scene. Yet, adequately supervised, the last look can afford the staff an opportunity to help the distressed, insistent family member gain composure. If they appear to be going to pieces, less insistent family members may be talked out of taking a last look.

Another decision that must be made about the family's last look is how long it will last and where it will take place. In the United States, the hospital viewing is usually expected to last only a few moments, to be taken up later in the funeral home. The family member who breaks down, then, can be whisked out of the room to control the scene. The family can take its last look anywhere in the hospital without threatening the sentimental order too much, although the staff may think twice about permitting it on an open or crowded ward where even brief crying is disturbing to many. Also, in only a few moments on an ICU or an emergency ward, a family member can knock over precious equipment. If the risk of a scene is great, the body may be moved to a private or treatment room for the viewing; or it may take place in the hospital morgue or autopsy room.

In Asia the last look may be considerably longer; in Japan, for example, it may be many hours. Since in these hospitals patients often die on open wards, the potential for disturbing scenes is great. In Japan, a post-mortem room (in the basement or on the grounds) is provided for the whole family and the body until the following day; thus the affair is isolated from everyone. In Malaya, a Chinese family just floods the open ward and wails at least ceremoniously, while an Indian family may take its last look on the ward and then repair to the courtyard to cry and moan.

The number of people involved is also an important consideration for averting scenes. In the United States, only a few close family members typically are allowed to see the body at the hospital. The remainder of the family and friends must wait until the undertaker has prepared the body. American hospitals, therefore, can become chaotic when a foreign person dies and his entire family, following their home custom, invades the ward for a last look. We learned of an extreme situation that arose when an Italian Gypsy queen died in a county hospital; not only her family but hundreds of her followers piled into the ward for a last look. The staff had no ready strategy to handle such a disturbance. In some Japanese hospitals, however, the whole family may come for the last look, but there is no problem because they are isolated in the patient's room. In Asia and Europe the ward may simply have to put up with many grief-stricken family members.

Also related to the "scene potential" is the presentability of the patient. This factor has an inverse relationship with the family's "need" for an after-death last look: relatives of quick-dying patients are more likely to request last looks after death, but less likely to be prepared for the fact of death. Patients who have had quick deaths are often more dreadful to view than others are. The causal accident or seizure often disfigures; the consequent heroic treatment often compounds the unpleasantness.

Viewing bodies of lingering patients who have withered away or whose bodies have partly degenerated can also be devastating to kinsmen; but, since post-death viewing is less common in these cases, and since kinsmen have been aware of dying's toll, it poses fewer problems.

Mode of death thus compounds the problem of preventing scenes during last looks. When an awesome mode of death makes the patient unviewable by the uninitiated, the doctor or nurse usually tries to talk the relative out of a last look. They almost routinely do so, for example, with parents of premature babies. If the mother never saw it alive, nurses maneuver to prevent a last look, usually by saying firmly that "it's just as well" she not see it. If the mother or father insists, the doctor is called to counsel strongly against it. With surgical deaths, when the body is mutilated, the doctor advises the family to wait until the body is prepared at the funeral home. He suggests that the relative would probably prefer to "remember him as he was," and the relative usually acquiesces, particularly when assured that the patient died peacefully, which gives the relative an imaginary or symbolic last look. In the case of accidents, which have a high scene potential if the body is mutilated, the strategy is to remove it to the hospital morgue or to the coroner as fast as possible. Prompt removal precludes a last look. As one nurse said when the relatives arrived on a county emergency ward, "They want to see him, so you'd better get him out of here in a hurry." Faced with a fait accompli, the relatives must wait until they can view the body at the funeral home.

In effect, when the mode of death is too unpleasant to allow the relative a last look, the hospital staff provides relatives a "symbolic" last look. In the case of preemies, mothers are left to their idealized images of babies. In the case of accident, surgical or other intensive-care cases, the relatives are asked to remember their best image of the person until they view him at the funeral home (where experts attempt to recreate this image). For these relatives, the mystic gap between life and death is closed symbolically. This may make the gap harder to grasp at the moment, but eases the threat to the ward's sentimental order posed by a potential hysterical scene.

When the relative does have a last look, the mystic gap may be closed more realistically—but sometimes more harshly. To ease the harsh reality when the mode of death has disfigured the body, the staff makes an effort to make it more presentable. They try to make the patient appear as the relatives might "remember him." They put a smile on his face to replace a grimace of pain. They dress him in fresh pajamas or even in street clothes. They hide, bandage, or disguise mutilated or severely damaged parts of the body that would be exposed. A chaplain reported of a surgical death that he "stalled and handled the relatives while the doctor went out and fixed the body just the way the body is sometimes fixed in the funeral parlor, and they put something on the patient's head so he wouldn't look so bloody." The staff may also remove the body from a surgical or emergency ward to an empty room in order to help "neutralize" the viewing. Sometimes staff insist that relatives who have requested a last look take it before the autopsy, in case the body is further disfigured beyond repair at the funeral home.

All in all, then, the patient's presentability is a temporally organized phenomenon that occurs quickly within the routines of the hospital. The staff has only a short time to fix up the body and to allow a last look before it is removed to the morgue, autopsy room, or funeral home. Seldom will they keep a body on a ward for hours while a family comes from afar for a last look; the delay would be too disturbing for the staff and too intrusive on needed hospital space.

The patient's appearance is also of concern to family members wishing to protect other, more upset members from a last look. A strong relative sometimes forbids a weaker one from seeing the body, particularly when damage or distortion is great. The strong member immediately, in trying to protect the living, makes and enforces the decision. In one such case, a daughter discovered her father's death upon arrival at the hospital; although surprised, she immediately recovered her control. Once the fact of death was established, her immediate reaction was, "I'll go catch mother." She intercepted her approaching mother in the hall, asserted that there was no point in her going into the patient's room, and sent her home with assurances that she would handle all details.

THE LAST TOUCH AND USHERING

The last look also presents a control problem beyond that of maintaining composure. The person who ushers in or escorts the relative must be able to handle a relative's need for a last touch— a none-too-easy task. Touching the body is part of relatives' effort to help close the mystic gap between life and death. It is typical for the relative at first to stand silently with disbelief and just look at the body. As the realization of death seeps in he touches it. The touch may be highly charged, may trigger highly emotional outbursts. In one instance reported to us, parents grabbed hold of their child and cried, "He's not dead, he's not dead," as they hugged and hugged the small boy. The nurse, a practiced "usher," was able to dislodge them after fifteen minutes. In another case, a daughter buried her face in her dead father's neck; the nurse could not free her and an orderly was called to help tear the girl loose. Thus, the mystic gap between life and death was forcefully closed. In another instance, a boy became hysterical on viewing his dead father, tore the cushions from the chairs, beat his fists on the walls, then grabbed the body and would not let go. He screamed, "You killed my father, he can't be dead." Again the nurse had to call for help. A chaplain, in this case, "talked" the boy away; by talking, the mystic gap closed. The doctor then gave him a sedative.

Happily, many last touches are gentle and moving, bringing to both the relative and the usher a modicum of composure—and perhaps closure. The relative may kiss the body, stroke the cheek, caress the hands, run hands through the hair, touch all the face areas. These touches seem to be a matter of assuring oneself that "everything is in place"; and thus they help close the mystic gap. Such a final, formal farewell is made even more real by touching a body that is still warm. The relative realizes he is saying goodbye at the point of genuine departure. The staff member watches and waits for the right moment, when the disbelief in death disappears, then gently ushers the relative out and takes him back to the family group.

The usher for these delicate situations often is a nurse who has a demonstrated flair for handling herself and family members. But others, too, may serve: a clerk, social worker, doctor, resident, aide, chaplain, nun. By and large however, personnel adept at ushering are relatively rare, and the task itself is sometimes not well understood. On one ward a head nurse was so unnerved by the last-look situation that she would not allow even capable nurses to usher in relatives. Rather than preserving the ward's sentimental order, her prohibition jolted it, for the nurses "felt the family should have an opportunity to see the body just to *realize* that the patient was really dead." Moreover, the relatives' closure of the mystic gap concerns the nurses also, because it helps reinforce their own closure on the death.

THE LAST DETAILS

After the last look, the family members still must settle details of the death with the hospital and gather up the patient's personal effects. At this point, the procedures for disposing of the family slow down. The announcement of death, the last look, and the last touch necessarily occur quickly in U.S. hospitals because the body is to be removed within a few hours after death. After disposition of the body, however, the staff must retain the family to handle the details of death, and therefore must slow down its departure. The standard strategy is to give sedation to the particular family members who must remain for a time. Besides reducing their pain of grieving and potential scenes in hallways and wards, this strategy allows the staff to deal with relatives who otherwise could not discuss such details as bills, an autopsy (if advisable), personal effects, and burial. The strategy helps staff and relatives to deal matter-of-factly with a highly emotional situation.

In some situations, the family either does not need to remain or is too slow in departing, to the annoyance of staff. For example, in emergency wards, if a patient dies before admittance or is dead on arrival, the only decision a relative must make is what to do with his kinsman's clothes. Never having been formally a patient, the body is not technically within the hospital's jurisdiction; the coroner takes charge and makes decisions with relatives. Thus the family can be removed quickly from the ward, with or without the patient's clothes. Sometimes the coroner must keep the personal effects for a time. In any case, the relative leaves directly after the last look. At the other extreme, the mother of a premature baby who has died may remain a patient for some time after the body has been sent to the funeral home. Her presence may itself be upsetting to staff; if she broods about the death, or wishes always to talk about it, the staff may become oversolicitous or antagonistic. A mother once wanted help from the nurses in naming a dead baby. This was very disturbing to the sentimental order of the word; the staff avoided such talk with her and wished she would be sent home. In an even more distressing case, a mother of a preemie who died returned six months later, looking for a baby to care for!

In any event, only the strongest family member, if there is is more than one at the hospital, needs to stay. This person is not necessarily an intimate relative, and can even be a distant one. The strongest is likely to be a man. "It's a man's world," one nurse explained when a "wastrel" son was retained for handling details, although the daughter had cared for the patient during his last ten years, and the nurse felt the daughter should have had more to say about the autopsy and burial arrangements.

Under other conditions, there are different strategies for slowing down the departure of relatives until the details are taken care of. In the case of lingering trajectories, relatives have very often largely finished their grieving before death. Details are handled as matter-of-factly as possible. The relative makes his rounds and decisions and leaves. When the relative is upset, a nurse may spend some time with him, talking calmly about the arrangements. The staff may give him coffee and show him to a private room so that he can relax for a time, requesting him to come out when he feels better. If the relative is extremely upset and will not take sedation, the staff may let him go home, asking him to come back the next day to see to details. But this is undesirable, because the signature on the forms signals the release of relatives; it is needed as soon as possible, especially for an autopsy. To release a relative before obtaining it creates difficulties in ultimately obtaining proper signatures.

This problem of dealing with an upset relative explains why the hospital may accept any relative's signature, as long as he is composed enough to know what he is signing. Finding the strongest relative, and getting rid of the rest, can be virtually impossible when several close relatives make claims to handling the details. We observed each of five grown children of an Italian mother, all of them upset, wishing to take care of things. Despite the confusion, the clerk wisely let all of them handle details, and in doing so they straightened each other out. The nurse said, "They all behaved much better when they were all together." Two fainted and the rest took care of them. If this strategy had not worked, however, handling the five family members would have been more difficult. By and large, dealing with several kinsmen poses a calculated risk to the sentimental order of the ward and to the processing of after-death details.

Another general strategy, with many variations, is the use of "escort services" to handle the family from the time of the death announcement until the details are finished. The service may be run by a chaplain, nun, social worker, ward clerk or nurse, or "details clerk." Chaplains and nuns are particularly adept at calming down relatives; they may take relatives to the chapel (if there is one) to pray and quiet down. The most objective escort service we observed was managed by the details clerk in a veterans hospital. This clerk's impersonality was based on having had no contact with the family before the death; her taking over the management of details dissociated the procedure from personnel whom the family associated with the death. Such an arrangement offers relief to the staff as well as momentary detachment to kinsmen. One nurse explained when asked how her geriatric hospital handled relatives of the dead: "Oh, 'details' handles that. We just send them down to 'details.' " This nurse had no idea of what "details" did, and was evidently glad to be uninvolved.

The details clerk we observed did little to handle the feelings of the relative. She just matter of factly asked about autopsy, funeral and cemetery arrangements, clothes, government and veterans benefits, and eye-bank donations. She did this in a special office containing a waiting couch, a setting suited to neutralizing and instrumentalizing the occassion. If relatives objected to an autopsy, she called in the doctor who wanted it, and had him talk to the family. So matter of fact (or jaded) are these clerks that one said of relatives, "They come in to see what they can get out of it [the death]," referring to gains from veterans benefits. Her lack of expressive support and her totally businesslike manner structure the interaction into a completely mechanical handling of details—a strategy that works, however intimidating it is to the relative.

Returning the personal effects of the dead patient is sometimes a very delicate situation; it may constitute a symbolic last look and therefore can precipitate another breakdown of the family member. Recognition of this symbolic potential can also be disturbing to the nurse who returns the clothes and other personal effects and to others on the ward who witness the occasion. The nurse can return these articles either directly or through others (details clerk, mortician, chaplain, or "the front desk"); the way she chooses depends upon several conditions.

A nurse who has had little or no previous contact with the family is likely to return the effects directly. Unlike the nurse who may have developed some involvement through previous contacts with the family, one who has had no contact is relatively immune to the family's grief. She may be able to accomplish the task bluntly and may wait until the best time, depending on her own ability to handle herself and the family. Moreover, with a relatively unknown nurse, the family is forced to stifle its grief during the ceremony, whereas with a known nurse they more easily give way to grief and tears. The unknown nurse clearly is less apt to meet questioning or accusations about the death; whereas taking personal effects from a known staff member provides one more occasion for the family to start questioning about how comfortably the trajectory ended. An unknown nurse also will seldom be asked to "make sense" of the death to the relative. The known nurse who wants to, and who feels her composure is up to it, may return these effects; but if both nurse and family member start to shed tears, the ward is disturbed. The known nurse therefore usually tries to be backstopped by a clerk, another nurse, or an aide who can help bring the scene to a close and reinstate the ward's sentimental order.

By and large, nurses do recognize the direct returning of personal effects as another opportunity for helping family members close the mystic gap between life and death. But since it can also be another opportunity for rehashing the death scene, some nurses routinely choose the indirect way; others use this method when the situation is especially highly charged. If the family member insists on getting personal items before leaving, the nurse may have to return them directly. But the kinsman's request takes the burden from her, since she is now complying with a request, not initiating the giving of the effects to an unsuspecting relative. In one coroner's case, on an emergency ward, a daughter asked if her father's body "still had the ring and watch." The coroner said, "He does, but I will have to get them for you because we have to record this information." "Thank you, I would like them tonight," said the daughter. The coroner, whose legal right it was to keep these effects, seized upon this insistence to have them as a tactic of keeping calm a daughter, who had been uncontrollably crying, so he could obtain further details from her on the death for his records.

After the relatives take care of the last detail concerning the patient's death at the hospital, they usually leave without further ceremony. However, sometimes they are escorted to the main entrance by a staff member. This happens especially when the patient's death involved high social loss or when the family member had been given sedation and put to bed. In Japan, after a lengthy period in the grieving room and the settling of details, one or more hospital nurses may gather on the front steps and bow to the family as they leave—a ceremonial ending to the dying trajectory. Uusually with the last detail finished—say, paying the hospital bill in an office near the lobby—the dying trajectory in the hospital is abruptly over for the American family.

DISPOSING OF THE BODY

Hospitals have made the disposal of the body routine in several ways. None is free of social-psychological hazards for the staff, though, mostly because of two problems. The body must be prepared according to proper procedures: who on the staff is to do it? The body must be removed as soon as possible to the hospital morgue or pathology laboratory (or funeral room in Italy or grieving room in Japan): while moving the body how does the designated staff member prevent the sight from disturbing other patients, their family members, and other staff members? Both of these questions pertain to the central issue of maintaining the sentimental order of the ward.

As we have mentioned, the body is supposed to be prepared and removed as soon as possible. Quick disposal removes death and the associated family from the ward, thus reducing the threat of disturbance to the sentimental order. The procedures that hospitals have developed to expedite the disposition are susceptible to interruption under unusual circumstances, as when an inquiry into the death is required. In one situation we encountered, for example, a nighttime suicide halted the usual order of disposition in several wards. The patient's doctor could not be reached, and on his way to the hospital the husband got caught in a traffic jam. Although an intern was roused to make the pronouncement, it was thought that the regular doctor should see the suicide situation before disposition of the body. Since it was a suicide, the question was raised as to whether the coroner had to see the body before it could be moved. The coroner could not be reached until morning. Therefore, the staff held the body on the ward for several hours, a delay that was very disturbing to the sentimental order.

In an instance of possible criminal abortion, it was not possible to move the body of the woman from the ICU, for the coroner must see the place where such a patient dies. "Oh, it was something," a nurse reported. "The supervisor was quite upset, didn't know whether we could move the body because she wasn't sure it was a coroner's case or not, because if it is a coroner's case, you aren't supposed to touch anything." So the coroner had to come to make the decision as to whether it was his case. By the time he arrived the body was in rigor mortis, which compounded the nurses' distress: "It looked pretty awful." Meanwhile, the girl's father, who would have missed it arrived and asked for a last look at his daughter, which was very upsetting for him and the nurses. Seldom will the ward staff hold up a disposition for the arrival of a relative; he can go to the morgue for a last look if the body is still in the hospital.

Sometimes it is not clear which ward is to dispose of the body. This problem arises when the patient is physically on one ward although technically assigned to another, or when death occurs while he is being moved. For example, if a patient is sent from the cancer ward to the ICU, and dies before he has been formally admitted, both wards may disclaim responsibility for disposal of the body. In one unique case, a patient on a medical ward jumped out of the window and was rushed to emergency, where he died before admittance. "The head nurse realized suddenly that she didn't have any precedent to go on. She didn't know what to do about this." First, she called the medical ward to come and get its patient. The medical resident came down and did the paper work on the emergency ward, but the body had to remain on the emergency ward several hours before the coroner arrived. In short, the medical ward handled the procedures for disposal of the body, but the emergency ward had to keep the body itself. As the medical ward did not call the coroner right away, the holding process was prolonged.

In extreme contrast, in one Italian hospital we found bodies sometimes disposed of immediately (no "wrapping"). For relatives without means, bodies are sent out of the hospital as if alive, in order for the record to indicate death at home. It is cheaper to move a supposedly live patient from the hospital by cab and then move him by hearse from home to the funeral. The hospital staff works with the family on this tactic, planning it before death (thereby taking the strain of disposal of a body off their own hands). In Italy we also found a geriatric ward which once kept bodies on the ward a whole day because of lack of manpower. This was highly demoralizing to other patients, who were forced for some hours into a morbid rehearsal of the end of their own trajectories and hospital careers.

Wrapping the body and otherwise physically preparing it for removal from the ward are routine but unwanted tasks. Generally, in America, they are done by a nurse, either one who is regularly assigned to them or the patient's own nurse. The preparations are usually done in the room in which the patient died, behind screens if there are other patients, or in the treatment room. On some wards, such as the premature baby ward, aides often are assigned this job, with a nurse checking their work. Many grumble at this task. In some instances, the task is delegated to student nurses—a gruesome learning experience that they hope will not be repeated.[1]

When nurses on other wards do not wish to prepare the body, they sometimes send it "alive" to the ICU, where it is admitted, discovered and pronounced dead, and wrapped. Staff on ICU's and emergency wards are watchful for this strategem. Another way to avoid wrapping the body, sometimes used by nurses on night shifts, is to draw curtains around the bed, as if the patient were sleeping, and let the next shift discover the body. A nurse

1. For many descriptive details on wrapping see David Sudnow, *Passing On* (pp. 77–90.)

said of this tactic, "It's really, really obnoxious. Here is this body sitting in bed for six hours, not wrapped, and there not five feet away a woman is sitting up eating breakfast. [Some nurses] feel they can get away with it."

In some Greek hospitals, nurses not only wrap the body, but also prepare it for burial and put it in a coffin. In Italian hospitals which have funeral rooms, the undertaker is part of the hospital staff, and he prepares the body. In the United States, nurses merely prepare the body for the hospital morgue, where the undertaker comes for it.

In their initial preparation of the body, American nurses initiate an important aspect of death mores, which continues both when the body is removed and at the funeral home. As nurses wrap the body in seclusion and prepare it for removal, they begin the suppression of all drama surrounding the death. The removal itself is done with as little drama and as little visibility as possible. The funeral director in his turn prepares the body for the appropriate dramas before burial—the wake, perhaps, and the funeral ceremony. In short, the hospital leaves *all* the drama of death up to the funeral director—its job is the care of the dying.

The effort to suppress all drama round the body has several consequences besides feeding into expressive drama guided by the funeral director. It is an act of control over the family members. It helps prevent them from making a scene by keeping them from viewing the body for too long; their last look may be only during a brief removal of the sheet from the kinsman's face. The tactic helps the family members save up their emotions for the funeral home, where they can express them freely. By helping to alienate the family from the body, the tactic serves to close the mystic gap and "grieve out" the kinsman. The nurses' work in disposing of the body is, therefore, consistent in several ways with the work of other people and organizations involved.

In order to achieve this suppression of drama, the nurse, in removing the body with the help of aides and orderlies, must work under varying ward conditions that may interfere with or help nonvisible disposals of bodies. Accordingly she develops, or the ward develops for her, strategies for nonvisible disposals that use the particular conditions that help or that prevent other conditions from converting disposals into a "public spectacle."

Wards vary in their potential visibility concerning the removing of bodies. On some wards disposition is within full view of everybody, because of the structure of the ward and the on-going activity on it. For example, on open wards in Asia and Europe, where they may be as many as 120 patients, there are many deaths, and all witness the removal of the covered corpse. This can create pandemonium among patients. In one such incident during the Christmas season, when a patient died unexpectedly, the nurses started the patients singing carols in order to bring them under control. On these wards, some patients panic after such a scene, leaving the hospital, and as a result die sooner.

In the United States, the most crowded wards, with the poorest layout for nonvisible removals, generally are emergency wards, especially those at city and county hospitals. On one ward we observed, bodies were carried past several patients and their relatives in the waiting area. On another emergency ward, the body has to travel 500 feet through public corridors and down a public elevator to the basement, with patients and relatives lining each side of the corridor. The disposition of the body under these conditions is like a "funeral procession." As concealment is impossible, the nurses must use strategies such as making the corpse "look alive" by leaving the sheet off the face—if they make any attempt at all at nonvisibility.

If the hospital rule is to remove the body immediately, regardless of how many people are around, ICU's and medical wards may have a similar problem. For example, at one veterans hospital where this was the rule, there were no waiting rooms, so the corridors were sometimes lined with visiting relatives and patients. Removal of a body provided a vivid rehearsal of death. Sometimes, to relieve the tension, the nurses would remove the sheet from the face and mumble, "He's going to X-ray." Also they tried to move the gurney rapidly in order to reduce the time that any one viewer could observe it.

Which patients actually watch a removal from the ward depends considerably, to be sure, on individual factors. But there are discernible tendencies. When the removal is a rehearsal for the patient's probable future—if he has a similar disease, particularly if it is far advanced—he is likely to turn away or return to his room and close the door. Thus he tries to suppress the drama that reminds him of his own fate. Similarly, a patient close to possible death for whatever reason also tends to avoid viewing a removal. But patients at earlier stages of a similar trajectory tend to view the removal with ambivalent curiosity, vaguely realizing that this might happen to them if they become worse. Patients with a clearly different illness trajectory and recovering patients generally watch the procession and the drama with only generalized involvement.

Most wards, however, can provide conditions that allow a nonvisible removal if the staff arranges it skillfully. Let us look at the general removal process in which strategies are linked to the layout of the ward. The first step is to remove the patient, if possible, before death to a private room or a room with privacy (for instance, a treatment room). When death occurs, the wrapping of the body is done without being observed or heard by other patients. If this is not possible, the dying patient's bed will be screened off, which prevents only observation, since other patients can still hear. If they ask what it is all about, they may be told a story such as "She is being prepared for X-ray." One patient, when hearing the story, retorted, "X-ray, hell, she's been dead for an hour." The nurse remained mute and upset and whisked the gurney out—the drama had broken through.

The next step is to get the body from the room to the elevator without being seen. Before this is begun, a call is put through to the morgue or pathology laboratory to alert its personnel to receive the body when the elevator lands. After this O.K., the nurses choose their time in the hallway; to make the way clear, they usually must wait until visiting hours are over, and close the doors to other patients' rooms. Then the elevator is stopped and the door held open by a nurse. The body, which is now covered by a sheet, is wheeled quickly by an orderly or aide to the elevator, put into it while the nurse dashes in behind it with her "forms" and closes the door.

If the hospital does not have work elevators, the nurses then must deal with the problem of a public elevator that anyone might stop. They may put an "out-of-order" sign on the elevator. If the elevator is stopped, they may refuse to let anyone in, or remove the sheet so that the body looks asleep, or work the buttons so that no entry is possible. Once in the basement, the body is quickly put in the morgue; and the removal is over, with there having been little or no visibility.

When the coroner removes a body from the ward, additional hazards may arise. Coroners' removals seem to vary from the extremely noisy, when staff members have to remind his orderlies to be quiet and discreet, to the highly polished, which are barely noticed even by the staff. For the staff, any drama inherent in even a noisy removal is overshadowed by their work with the living and by their release from the task of removing the body. (We were not told if the patients or relatives noticed the removal.) However, before one such removal, two ambulance drivers were suppressing the drama surrounding a dead-on-arrival patient while waiting for the police and coroner to arrive. They stood guard over the room where the body was, to prevent entry, and acted as if something were going on inside that would save the patient. They called this "babysitting" and warded off other patients who might be put in the room, or relatives who might arrive to see the patient.

DISPOSITION OF THE PATIENT'S STORY

After the body and family are gone from the ward, there remains only the staff's disposition of the patient's story among themselves. This disposition is a social-psychological process that brings the story of the patient's dying and death to a close in their minds. The degree to which it is necessary varies. At one extreme are the stories of patients whose dying trajectories and deaths were typical and expected. These stories are routine and never really bothersome; since they were accurate before death, there is no need to develop post-mortem stories. When these patients have been removed from the ward, they tend simply to be forgotten by the staff.

But several kinds of patients have had while dying a strong or unusual story that is difficult to forget, and some have had an inaccurate pre-death story, or none at all. The kind of disease or condition a patient died from may have bewildered the staff, may have been unknown, or "very interesting," or "awful," or a complete surprise. In short, some characteristics of the conditions of death or the disease may generate a need for a post-mortem story about the patient. This story explains what happened and is part of the staff's bringing the case to a close and, in effect, "erasing" it from the sentimental order of the ward. Characteristics of the patient himself (he had a high social loss, was mentally ill, was obnoxious, had a "wonderful personality" while facing death) and characteristics of the family or one of its members (a young widow and children were left destitute, a son had a mother who would not visit him) also help generate a post-mortem story about the patient. The two principal factors in bringing the story to a close are the autopsy findings and the staff's discussion among themselves and with relatives. Staff members also may have to come to terms with the patient's story through personal grieving and introspection. Often all three ways are combined.

Talk develops the post-mortem story; it is largely a reconstruction of the dead patient's dying story and what staff did during the case. If the dying story was inaccurate, it is reconstructed in terms of the signs that were missed in order to determine now why staff's handling of the case went awry—as in a suicide or other surprise death—or why staff expected something different. The post-mortem story explains what really happened and if necessary "absolves" the personnel of negligence, while teaching them what to look for next time. For its fullest possible development, the post-mortem story may require an autopsy. If there was no story on a patient—*e.g.,* he was dead on arrival—its development now is simply an effort to clarify what happened.

The post-mortem discussion may cover a wide range of topics. Two questions that often are debated, especially in cases with lingering trajectories, are, "Did he know he was dying?" and, "Did he die in pain?" The awareness question arises when a patient, who was never told he was dying but had plenty of time to discover it, neither indicated explicitly that he had done so nor put his affairs in order or otherwise prepared himself. This apparent lack of awareness can be disturbing to nurses, and after death they may regret it. Hence they often debate whether he really did know and privately prepared himself and whether his unawareness may have been pretense. The question of pain arises in lingering illnesses when the patient cannot talk or is comatose at the end, for pain management is harder; whether the patient died in comfort is debatable. As a way of establishing for themselves whether they were negligent or helpless in providing a comfortable death, nurses frequently debate whether they gave enough sedation at the end. In quick trajectories, pain and awareness are less at issue, for time is taken up with intense work and the patient is often unconscious from the start of the trajectory.

Another feature that often generates extended development of the post-mortem story among nurses is a unique death that provides them with possible dying rehearsals for their own fates. In one poignant case, a nurse died following an illegal abortion. This was quite disturbing to other nurses, who thought, among other things, that a nurse should know better. They discussed at length how this could have happened to their former colleague, and how it could happen to them, even though they did "know better." Death from breast cancer also has a high story potential.

High social loss cases tend to be explained along lines of a general rationale that it is better that the patient died. Although his loss was high, his condition would have made further living unbearable or useless: "He was no loss to anyone when he was that bad off."

Dead-on-arrival cases tend to generate story development about what could have happened and about the patient's real medical condition and history. If the person is from Skid Row, police are asked for records. Wallets are scanned for names of relatives or doctors who can give information. When ambulance drivers bring in a DOA, acting as if they were keeping him alive with oxygen because they cannot pronounce him dead, doctors ask the drivers when he stopped breathing. They try to pin down the real story, not the incomplete or fictional one created until a doctor pronounces death. Drivers and nurse may then go on to talk about how they go through similar situations, "three times a day." In the case of the cancer patient who jumped out of the window and was brought dead to the emergency ward, there was much talk about whose patient he was, who was to dispose of him, and the general problem of jurisdiction and responsibility posed by the story. Car accidents and fights ending in death also generate stories imbued with "their own fault" theories about why the patients died.

The surprise quick trajectory typically raises two topics for staff discussion: "Was anyone negligent?" and "What was the stress on the person who found the body?" Sometimes staff members hold a formal meeting to discuss why a surprise death occurred. As they piece together what they did and did not do or notice, they continually must handle the implied and subtle accusations of negligence arising among them: "I guess there isn't much we could do because all these things we have been talking about could happen to other patients, too, you know." They also console each other for mistakes. Mostly they realize that they are not being held accountable for the many acts that could have been different, *e.g.*, reporting indicators of potential suicide. Any feelings of negligence about discounting, through ignorance or lack of understanding, what should not have been discounted and might have been prevented, are relieved. Moreover, autopsy may show that death—say, on the operating table—occurred because of a condition that no one could have foreseen. Autopsies may, therefore, sometimes be urged on the family in order to resolve the story for the staff.

Following a surprise death, there may be a constant interweaving of work loss and social loss in the patient's story. These themes are particularly important when the dead person was someone—a wife with children, for example—who "should have been" saved because of her importance to others. In one case of work loss, a doctor performed 25 operations to restore the face of a man who toward the end of his ordeal committed suicide. In talking about it the doctor said, "You know, it makes me wonder, could I have been more sympathetic?" Though he was not held accountable for social-psychological negligence but only for the medical work, which was done to perfection, the effort he had put into his work affected his feelings about the former.

The staff member who finds the body of a completely unexpected, surprise death usually must be comforted by colleagues, and a post-mortem story ensues. If the story development does not calm the nurse or aide, she may have to be transferred to another ward to reduce her memories. In one case, a nurse went into a prolonged discussion about how "it is one thing to walk into a room, and how horrible it is to find somebody dead and particularly to find an object you are not used to in one way like this, with her tongue hanging out and all that, really pretty messy." The nurse or aide who found the body usually talks about it also with intimates other than her colleagues, in the attempt to "work through" her own feelings.

The post-mortem story is mainly an informal one, developed within the ward until it is forgotten. However, sometimes the manner of death is so momentous, especially with surprise quick trajectories, that the story breaks through the boundaries of the ward itself. If the patient had been on several wards, news of a surprise or "ugly" death may travel in shock waves throughout the hospital. The news travels through questions and answers "on the grapevine." As the news resounds through the hospital corridors, the story becomes formalized and pared down so that it can be passed along faster. In the surprise suicide or table death, the story may become further formalized by a coroner or through an inquest, and perhaps then be picked up by the newspapers and spread through the community or nation.

Sometimes, if the death story reaches the newspapers, and investigations by outside agencies are started, the hospital comes into question. For example, in a hospital which had a rule that when all beds were occupied no more patients could be admitted, a man was turned away from the emergency ward and died for lack of care. A staff member surreptitiously reported the incident to the newspapers, hoping that public revelation would put the hospital administration under pressure to be more flexible. Frequently, when this sort of post-mortem story gets into the newspaper, while putting the hospital's organization in view, it also brings other organizations or systems that partially caused the death under public scrutiny; for example, a factory, prison, or bus system.

Several properties of the post-mortem story, as developed by staff in the effort to dispose of these "remains" of the patient, are important for us to note. The staff are as focused on completing the disposition as on the reality behind it. The day and evening staff is usually more involved in the after-death story than the night staff, because of their greater involvement in the living story of the patient. A suicide at night provides an exception. Further, there is usually no formal mechanism for formulating a post-mortem story. Sometimes, however, it develops as the byproduct of a routine staff conference. Or, if the ward's sentimental order is in disarray—as from the unexpected deaths of three adolescents within a few days—and does not seem to be recovering fast enough, the head nurse may call a special conference. In one case, a head nurse asked a psychiatrist to preside over the discussion.[2] But by and large, discussions in the corridors and nursing stations, combined with the press of work and new stories, finally put each post-mortem story to rest.

Another important feature of the post-mortem story is its description of the temporal aspects of the patient's trajectory, which we call "time-jamming" and "time-spreading." As personnel review the case they may jam months of lingering into a few moments of discussion and spread out a few strategic moments of the trajectory into a detailed 20-minute discussion of, say, what everyone was doing when the patient's tubes fell out without notice. Time-jamming and time-spreading indicate the relevant parts of the pre-death story that have bothered the staff. Subsequently, the story is steered purposively, if unwittingly, in a clearly negative or positive manner so as to balance out sentimentally what happened. As we have mentioned earlier, in a death with high social loss, for example, the "negative" story is likely to be developed to show that it was best he died, since he could no longer have a useful life. In an accident case, the negative story may be developed to indicate that it was the driver's "own fault" and that, although the death is a tragedy, he got what he deserved. For a suicide, the staff may develop a "positive" story— that everyone has a right to decide when to end his own life. In the case of older people, the positive story may hinge around how full a life they have had.

When a post-mortem story cannot be clearly slanted in order to provide the needed balancing, to justify in the staffs' minds what actually happened, then the patient's story may linger on in the minds of nurses for months. These cases become unforgettable. Whenever we asked nurses and aides to tell us about a death, these were the cases remembered first. Obviously they still needed to talk about them. When the sentimental order of the ward recovers after such a case, many nurses must dispose of the per-

---

2. This tactic did not help too much since he steered the discussion away from the kind of dying that nurses know about and wanted to mull over "guilt feelings," which did not mean much to staff.

sisting "remains" on a personal level. They do not discuss the case openly with colleagues, again because of the potential disturbance of the ward's sentimental order. They may remember certain deaths, because of their personal reactions, for many years.

Perhaps the most positive story—and most biased description of a death—is the "perfect image of death" that nurses and doctors sometimes give family members who have missed the death scene and a last look. They give such a story even when the death was gruesome and the patient obnoxious. For example, premature babies may be ugly at death, cancer patients are often in a deteriorated condition, and some patients swear and yell at the staff. In one extreme example, a fat woman who was an alcoholic fell into a bathtub of hot water and scalded herself. Her smell was particularly repugnant to nurses, and they thought her accident was her "own fault." After her death, they told her closest relative that she liked to have a drink or two, had a fainting spell, fell in the bath and had a stroke, "poor thing." "Why beat the dead?" was the response to our question of why not tell the relative what happened and how she died.

There are several reasons for such stories. It is difficult to tell an uncomfortable story to a relative; such a story might also cause the family to create a scene. More important, perhaps, nurses often feel that the relative has been denied rightful participation in the death, and therefore needs this vacuum to be filled with a story. They fill it with eulogy based on images of a "perfect death" in comfort and peace. The family member leaves the hospital with a comforting, peaceful story to take him through the following months. It makes the nurses feel better, too.

XI

Time, Structural Process, and Status Passage

In our opening pages, we remarked that the temporal features of work are of the utmost importance for understanding how organizations function. On virtually every page of this book, readers have found materials pertinent to the temporal features of work organizations and trajectories. Now those features will be discussed within the more general context of the sociology of time.

It is useful to begin by thinking of the hospital career provided for a dying trajectory as a succession of "transitional statuses" in the status passage between life and death,[1] as it takes place in the hospital. In contrast to Wilbert Moore's concepts[2] of sequence, rate, synchronization, rhythm, routines and recurrence, which simply denote time unrelated to social structure, transitional status is a concept denoting *social structural* time. How does a social system keep a person in passage between two statuses for a period of time? He is put into a transitional status, or a sequence of them, that denotes a period of time during which he will be in a status passage (*e.g.*, he is put on the ICU, thereby denoting a quick passage). As a concept for ordering social structural time, transitional status has great advantages over Moore's concepts. His concepts help us talk of the social ordering of behavior; but they are not automatically linked with social structure; they are only

1. Glaser and Strauss, "Temporal Aspects of Dying as a Non-Scheduled Status Passage," *American Journal of Sociology*, Vol. 71 (1965), pp. 48–59.
2. See *Man, Time and Society* (New York: John Wiley, 1963), Chapter 1.

applied to it, if the analyst is so inclined. In contrast, referring to the transitional statuses of a status-passage, on the other hand, automatically requires locating the discussion within a social structure.

In general, sociological writing about groups, organizations and institutions tends to leave their temporal features unanalyzed.[3] When they are handled explicitly, the focus is on such matters as deadlines, scheduling, rates, pacing, turnover, and concepts of time which may vary by organizational, institutional or group position. The principal weakness of such analyses stems from an unexamined assumption that the temporal properties worth studying involve only the work of organizations and their members. For instance, the work time of personnel must be properly articulated —hence deadlines and schedules. Breakdowns in this temporal articulation occur not only through accident and poor planning, but also through differential valuation of time by various echelons, personnel and clientele. But from our analysis the temporal order of the organization appears to require much wider range of temporal dimensions. We have assumed in this book that, for instance, people bring to an organization their own temporal concerns and that their actions there are profoundly affected by those concerns.[4] Thus, woven into our analysis were experiential careers (hospital, illness, and personal), as well as the patient's and the families' concepts of time. In our analysis, we have attempted to show how temporal order in the hospital refers to a total, delicate, continuously changing articulation of these various temporal considerations. Such articulation, of course, includes easily recognizable organizational mechanisms but also less visible ones, including "arrangements" negotiated by various relevant persons.

The kind of analysis required when studying temporal order brings our discussion to the two other topics of this chapter—

3. The following pages are adapted or quoted from the introduction to *George Herbert Mead on Social Psychology* ed. by Anselm Strauss, (Chicago: University of Chicago Press, 1964 edition), pp. xiii–xiv.

4. This kind of view is implicit in the writings of G. H. Mead. Herbert Blumer has attempted to make the view more explicit in his writing about Mead and in various papers about symbolic interactionism. *Cf.,* his "Society as Symbolic Interaction," in A. Rose (Ed.), *Human Behavior and Social Processes* (Boston: Houghton Mifflin, 1962), pp. 179–92.

structural process and status passage. Such a conception of how to study temporal order emphasizes the continual interplay of structure and process. Critics who incline toward a processual view of society have frequently criticized—and in our judgment effectively—the over-determinism of structuralists. But that critique need not necessitate an abandonment of the tremendously useful mode of thinking which is called "structural." That analytic mode need only be combined systematically with an allied concern with process. The study of dying trajectories within hospital organizations happens to have led easily to *thinking generally* about "structural process" and "status passage." Let us consider each in turn.

STRUCTURAL PROCESS

One of the central issues in sociological theory is the relationship of structure to process. What implication does this book have for this issue? We have, in previous chapters, discussed explicitly the structural adaptations of hospitals to various phases of dying trajectories. If one considers dying as a process extending over time, then the hospital's structure can be seen as continually changing to handle different phases in that process. Its structure, then, is in process; which phenomenon we call "structural process." We have seen how a person may be brought into one section of the hospital and then moved to another, as his trajectory is redefined or as he reaches certain critical junctures in an anticipated or defined trajectory. Even when a dying patient remains on one ward, he can be moved around within that ward so that different aspects of its "structure" can be brought into play. If he is never moved, the ward's or hospital's varying resources of manpower, skill, drugs or machinery may be brought into play as his trajectory proceeds. What is true for the staff's relationships with a patient is also true for its relationships with his family.

Sociological analysis ordinarily does not join structure and process so tightly as our notion of "structural process" does. Structure tends to be treated as relatively fixed—because it is what it is, then certain processes can occur. Or inversely, because the major goals involve certain processes, as in a factory or in a governmental agency, the structure is made as nearly consonant with the processes as possible. New processes are conceived as leading to new structural arrangements; while innovations in structure similarly lead to associated processual changes. A major implication of our book is that structure and process are related more complexly (and more interestingly) than is commonly conceived.

We have, for instance, remarked how during a given phase of a trajectory a ward may be quite a different place than before. For instance, when the sentimental order has been profoundly disrupted, the structural elements that can be called on are not quite the same as before; some elements no longer exist and may never again exist. If afterward an "equilibrium" is reached, it is a moving equilibrium with the ward calmed down but forever at least a somewhat different place.

So, rather than seeing a relatively inflexible structure, with a limited and determinable list of structural properties, we have to conceive of a ward, hospital, or any other institution as a structure in process. It therefore has a potential range of properties far greater than the outsider (the sociologist) can possible imagine unless he watches the insiders at work. He can be surprised at the ways in which staff, family or patients can call on diverse properties of the hospital or local community, for bringing in resources that he never dreamed existed but which became permanently or temporarily part of the structural processes of the ward.

In a previous work, one of the authors and his colleagues made a similar point, but neither gave it a name nor developed it as we are doing here.[5] It was remarked then that ordinarily state mental hospitals are conceived as places of limited resources, but that their personnel, when observed closely, exhibit great variation

5. Anselm Strauss *et al., Psychiatric Ideologies and Institutions* (New York: Free Press of Glencoe, 1965).

not only in how they use the obvious resources of the hospital but also in how they draw upon outside resources. If we interpret that latter set of operations in terms of structural process, we would say that the innovating personnel are making use of the to give lectures, or asks his own analyst to advise him, however in- outside resources (say, a young psychiatrist who asks colleagues directly, on how to handle his subordinates.) These resources are as much a part of the hospital "system"—at least for the time being—as anything found in the hospital itself. And they come into play during determinable times: they function neither independently of time nor of circumstance.

Perhaps we need especially to emphasize that the clients of an institution—patients or family members—are also structural features of it. Thus, a Japanese mother who cares for her dying son at a hospital becomes part of the hospital's structure. If the family gathers around during a patient's last days, then the hospital's structure is amplified. If families are banished or voluntarily "pull out" during certain phases of dying, then they do not loom large as structural possibilities for the staff to call on or to handle.[6]

Structural process relates to the various participants' awareness. They will vary, of course, in their awareness of which structural properties are operating, or can be brought to operate, during various phases of the dying process. Misperceptions are involved as well as awareness; a doctor, for instance, may assume that he can call on some structural resource (*e.g.*, an oxygen tank) when it no longer exists. He may discover its "disappearance" too late; or he may never discover his error, if it is not very consequential. Others, such as the nurses, may or may not be aware of the absence or presence of his knowledge. The relationships of these "awareness contexts" to structural processes are neither accidental nor unpredictable, as staff and patients sometimes believe.

Perhaps the point that most requires underlining, however, is

6. Herbert Simon makes the point that clients are as much part of an organization as its personnel, but he makes the point statically. See his *Administrative Behavior* (New York: Macmillan, 1948).

that structural process has consequences which themselves enter into the emergence of a *new* structural process. For the sociologist, this fact implies an important directive: part of his job is to trace those consequences that significantly affect the unrolling course of events called "structural process"—not for particular cases, but for *types* of cases. Sociologists, for instance, are not interested in *a* dying person, but in *types* of dying persons and the patterned events relevant to their dying. When focusing on the consequences of structure and process, it is all too easy to settle for lists of consequences for, say, various personnel or for the repetitive functioning of an organization or institution. But the explicit directive given by the concept of structural process is that the sociologist cannot rest until he has analytically related the interactional consequences to the next phases in interaction—or, in our terms, present structural processes to later structural processes.

THE DYING TRAJECTORY AS A STATUS PASSAGE

It is not necessary to review our substantive theory of dying trajectories, except to remind readers of several points: dying must be defined in order to be reacted to as dying; defining occurs not only at the beginning but throughout the courses of the various trajectories; hospitals are organized for handling various trajectories, including the establishment of specialized locales for handling different types of trajectories; work at those locales is organized in terms of a range of expected trajectories; a principal feature of these trajectories is the attempts by various parties to shape them; this shaping is affected by various cross-cutting variables (such as social loss, experiential careers and awareness); the various parties may differentially perceive the trajectories; the juggling of tasks, people and relationships during the course of anyone's dying opens possibilities for a considerable misalignment of actions that are usually quite well aligned. Our analyses have established that ascertainable structural conditions are related to the above items, and that their important consequences are also explainable—even somewhat predictable, provided one has advance knowledge of the relevant variables.

This substantive theory of dying trajectories has two especially valuable features. First, it is *dense:* it consists of a great number of propositions, so many indeed that the total theory is not easily summarized. One must almost read the book in order to grasp the theory in anything like its complex density. Second, the theory is *integrated:* the numerous propositions are related systematically to each other throughout our total discussion, and in complex fashion—and yet, we trust, with sufficient clarity to indicate the varying levels of abstractness at which they are formulated.

These two features—density and integration—contribute to the theory's *generality*. By this term, we mean that the theory is applicable to the multitude of diverse situations of dying trajectories. We remarked on this in our earlier book, *Awareness of Dying*.[7]

> Through the level of generality of our concepts we have tried to make the theory flexible enough to make a wide variety of changing situations understandable, and also flexible enough to be readily reformulated, virtually on the spot, when necessary, that is, when the theory does not work. The person who applies our theory will, we believe, be able to bend, adjust, or quickly reformulate . . . theory as he applies it in trying to keep up with and manage the situational realities that he wishes to improve."

This implies that the density, integration, and generality of the substantive theory increase the control that the user can obtain over various contingencies that may arise during the course of dying. To quote again:

> To give this kind of control, the theory must provide a sufficient number of general concepts and their plausible interrelations; and these concepts must provide him with understanding, with situational controls, and with access to the situation in order to exert the controls.[8]

7. *Awareness of Dying, op. cit.*, p. 265. For a general discussion of generality, density and integration see our *Discovery of Grounded Theory*.
8. *Op. cit.*, p. 268.

It scarcely seems necessary to emphasize that such control also stems from the "grounded" origins of the substantive theory: that is, the theory was not conceived prior to the research but evolved during it.

After a substantive theory is formulated, it is useful, when possible, to scrutinize its relationship to an existing formal theory. The aim is twofold: The scrutiny can lead to further formulation of the substantive theory; it can also lead to discovery and development of gaps in the formal theory. A dying trajectory, as we have suggested, can be usefully thought of as a type of *status passage:* the dying person is passing—through "transitional" statuses—between the statuses of being alive and being dead; various other participants are correspondingly involved with and implicated in his passage.[9]

The phenomena of status passages were enduringly called to the attention of sociologists and anthropologists by Van Gennep's *Rites du Passage.*[10] In that book, the French scholar remarked on various types of passages between what, in modern vocabulary, are termed "statuses." Mainly, he analyzed such passages as those which occur between age-linked statuses such as adolescence and adulthood, and between being unmarried and being married. Those kinds of passages have, of course, been very thoroughly studied since Van Gennep's day. Sociologists have also expended considerable effort in studying passages that occur within occupations ("socialization," for instance) and within organizations ("mobility," for instance). A principal characteristic of most of those passages is that they are governed by rather clear rules, bearing on when the passage should or can be made and by whom (scheduled); the sequences of steps that the person must go through to have completed the passage (prescribed steps); and what actions must be carried out by various participants so that the passage will actually be accomplished (regularized actions).

9. Cf. Glaser and Strauss, "Temporal Aspects of Dying as a Non-Scheduled Status Passage," *op. cit.*

10. Translated by M. Vizedom and G. Cafee (Chicago: University of Chicago Press, 1960). The original publication date was 1908.

These dimensions are so integral in numerous status passages that anthropologists and sociologists usually have focused on descriptions of the rituals—extremely scheduled, prescribed sequences of regulated actions—that tend to accompany at least certain phases of those passages.

Scheduling, regularization, and prescription are important dimensions of many, but not all, status passages. Each dimension can be absent, or present only to a degree. Furthermore, certain other relevant dimensions may characterize a type of passage. Thus, the passage may be considered (by the person making the passage or by other relevant parties) as in some measure *desirable* or undesirable. The passage may or may not be *inevitable*. It may be *reversible* and, if so, it may even be *repeatable*. The person undergoing the passage may do so *alone,* or *collectively* with any number of other persons of whose passages he may or may not be *aware*. Also, *clarity* of the signs of passage as seen by various people may be very great or very slight. The person making the passage may do so *voluntarily* or have no choice in the matter, have degrees of choice about varying aspects of it. Another dimension is the degree of *control* that various agents, including the central figure, have over various aspects, and during various phases, of the passage. One final dimension is especially noteworthy: the passage may require special *legitimation* by one or more agents.

Our research has shown the importance of distinguishing clearly among such structural dimensions of passage, and among their various possible permutations. When studying particular types of passage, the analyst could focus, according to their relevance, on several characteristic dimensions. Thus, Julius Roth has, without explicitly recognizing that recovery from severe TB can be conceptualized as a status passage, quite correctly emphasized the indeterminant pace of recovery, the ambiguity of signs of recovery as the patient sees them, and the patient's manipulations in getting his condition defined "upward" by the legitimating physician.[11] Similarly, when writing of degradation ceremonies,

11. *Timetables* (Indianapolis: Bobbs-Merrill, 1963).

Harold Garfinkel almost inevitably emphasized legitimacy: the degrading agent must manage to legitimate his activity and his role to make his accusation persuasive.[12] Orrin Klapp's analysis of how people are made into fools also had its appropriate focus: the successful or unsuccessful strategies of the foolmaker, and of the person who either manages or fails to avoid that status and who manages or fails to reverse the passage once cast into it.[13] To note one last example, Lloyd Warner's detailed description of an Australian tribe almost necessarily turned around a discussion of sequential and collective passages, carefully regulated so that entire segments of the tribe were involved at particular times and places.[14]

Analysis of a given status passage may be incomplete, however, if the social scientist focuses only on one, two or three relevant dimensions of the passage. It is also necessary that he trace the structural conditions under which passage is made, say, alone rather than collectively, or voluntarily rather than involuntarily. He must also research the consequences of these structural conditions for the various participants and the groups or institutions to which they belong—as well as their import for social interaction. A systematic analysis will also clarify the "exceptions"—that is, the variable patterns of interaction and consequence that occur when a normally important dimension is absent or modified. We cannot expect that these tasks can be accomplished unless the analyst is aware that his analysis can usefully be conceived as pertaining to status passages. If not, then he can be expected to make only a very incomplete analysis of his materials, with regard to status passages. Were this kind of analysis conscientiously attempted, it would be detailed, woven densely and quite lengthy. Of course, it is possible to analyze one or two dimensions systematically within a single journal article, but fuller analysis would

12. "Conditions of Successful Degradation Ceremonies," *American Journal of Sociology*, Vol. 61 (1956), pp. 420–24.
13. "The Fool as a Social Type," *American Journal of Sociology*, Vol. 55, (1949), pp. 159–60.
14. *A Black Civilization* (New York: Harper, 1937).

require much more space, perhaps as many pages as in this book.

The major dimensions of a dying trajectory as a status passage are unquestionably the ones noted earlier, in opposition to Van Gennep's discussions. First, dying is almost always *unscheduled;* second, the sequence of steps is *not institutionally prescribed;* and third, the actions of the various participants are only *partly regulated.* It is also quite relevant that the transitional statuses of dying (though not necessarily death itself when it comes) are usually defined as *undesirable.* Among the other relevant but highly variable dimensions are: the *clarity* of signs that are available to the various participants; the amount of *control* that the participants (including the patient) have over aspects of his passage; whether the passage is *traversed simultaneously* by multiple patients or whether only the patient is dying; and which, if any, patients in a simultaneous passage are *aware* of particular aspects of that process.

Complex permutations of those interrelated dimensions give rise, as we can now see, to the many variations of dying trajectories described earlier. This book could very well have been explicitly organized around the concept of status passage, with full focus on the systematic permutation of its dimensions. We chose not to write the analysis in that manner, for two principal reasons. First, the substantive theory eveloved during our research long before we understood its full relationship to a systematically formulated theory of status passages. Second (and more important, since we could have "converted" the substantive theory) we much preferred to present a substantive theory because of the infinitely greater sense of immediacy to dying situations that it would give our readers. After writing the book, we realized that a well-presented substantive theory would pass an especially critical test if it actually measured up to what a formal theory would require of it. When judged by that criterion, the substantive theory of trajectories measures up well. Unquestionably, however, something is lost when an analysis is not explicitly organized in accordance with a formal theory. For instance, some emphases in the "non-scheduling" paper are not at the foreground of analysis in the present book.[15]

It now seems to us that anyone who wishes to develop substantive theory about any phenomenon that might also be usefully seen as a status passage can considerably speed up his systematic guidance of research and his generation of substantive theory by a formal theory of status passage. But he must not do so too rigidly; he must avoid operating only within the framework of that formal theory—unless he is principally interested in the formal theory itself. Otherwise he runs the risk of radically closing off the possibilities of developing other aspects of substantive and formal theory. If we had, for instance, focused only (or principally) on status passage, we would not have developed the related substantive theory of awareness contexts. (Readers have seen it used, in crosscutting fashion, in this book.) Thus the total theory would have been more restricted in scope, less complex in its interrelationships, less dense, and certainly less widely applicable to dying situations.

To keep the record accurate, we should add that we began the research with two general ideas. One was that dying "took time," and thus was a process. The other idea, derived from personal experience, was that a collusive game of "evasion of the truth" often occurred around dying people. The second idea evolved organically into a theory of awareness contexts. The first idea evolved into a theory of dying trajectories long before we sensed its relevance to a theory of status passages. Therefore, we reiterate that formal theory should be used, but judiciously—and the earlier in the research it is used, the more wary the researcher should be of overcommitting himself to that formal theory.

When the substantive research is brought to a conclusion, what should it contribute to a preexisting formal theory? All too often, research based on (or brought into alignment with) a formal

15. Glaser and Strauss, "Temporal Aspects of Dying as a Non-Scheduled Status Passage," *op. cit.* See also *Discovery of Grounded Theory, op. cit.*, Part I, on relation between substantive and formal theory. On this, see also the introduction to Barney Glaser, *Organizational Careers* (Chicago: Aldine Publishing Company, 1968).

theory adds nothing to the theory; it merely applies it. Relevant substantive research, however, must elaborate, supplement, correct, critically test or in some other way stand in an instrumental relationship to the formal theory. Correspondingly, research that initiates a new substantive theory should lead to suggestions for the formulation and study of a related formal theory.[16]

Since it is our intention to present in another volume a formal theory which combines status passage and awareness context, we shall conclude the present discussion with two general remarks. First: the method used in discovering substantive theory—the systematic use of comparison groups—can be used effectively for generating a formal theory of a status passage.[17] The general procedure is to study simultaneously, or in quick succession, a number of kinds of status passages. The constant comparison of these will quickly draw attention to their many similarities and differences; the analysis generates the formal theory. Probably one need not engage in much firsthand gathering of data, for a number of status passages have been studied or described by social scientists. These materials can be used in "secondary analysis." So can the abundant popular material that an ingenious researcher can bend to his uses—for instance, books like *Diabetes as a Way of Life, Thank God for My Heart Attack, Managing Your Coronary, The Changing Years, What to Do about Your Menopause;* or materials on "getting ahead" in business, or "how to prepare" for motherhood or any other status; as well as such writings as the book in which John Griffin described how he, a white journalist, "passed" back and forth between the race lines in the Deep South, or the published autobiographies of con men which reveal clearly how they manage the status passages of their "marks." [18] Data represented by such publications can be used flexibly for building formal theory through constant comparisons, since the

16. For an example of this, see *Awareness of Dying, op. cit.,* pp. 276–80.

17. *Ibid.;* *The Discovery of Grounded Theory, op. cit.,* Chapters III and IV.

18. John Griffin, *Black Like Me* (Boston: Houghton Mifflin, 1960); cf. Edwin Sutherland, *The Thief* (Chicago: University of Chicago Press, 1937).

researcher will be guided by his evolving theory to either new uses of his data or the discovery of valuable new data.

A second point that deserves underscoring is that the same paradigm suggested earlier for substantive research about status passages can be used for developing formal theory about such passages. The theorist cannot be content with isolating and relating a few important dimensions of status passage. His theory must include their structural conditions, their interactional consequences (including relevant strategies), and their consequences for relevant participants and organizations. If this mandate is followed, the formal theory will be dense, integrated, of great scope and of considerable applicability. The theory will also be helpful in guiding new studies of status passages—as well as being useful in critical reviews of older studies.

XII

Improving the Care of the Dying

Our research has radical implications for changing, and perhaps improving, the nursing and medical care given to the dying. No reader can have read the foregoing chapters without drawing such conclusions, and assuredly many will have made further judgments about the terminal care that should and conceivably might be given. One can neither read or write such chapters without responding critically to what transpires in our hospitals. Yet we caution against too hasty a criticism of particular practices without considering them within a more comprehensive context, such as is represented by this book. Viewed within that context, some otherwise "senseless," "impersonal," "dehumanizing," or "ineffective" practice may be seen as the best alternative available under the conditions of any given time and place.

In our opening pages, we remarked on the striking trend toward the use of hospitals and allied institutions (like nursing homes) as the locales where people choose to die. This trend is consonant with the current importance of the hospital and its clinics as the central institution in the entire medical-care system. Even when relatively small, the modern hospital is a place where many professionals of diverse trainings and experiences work together in a complex division of labor, utilizing highly developed medical technology as they combat a multitude of diseases. In Western countries, where the incidence of serious infectious disease has greatly declined, hospital staffs are increasingly treating the acute phases of chronic illnesses. For those patients who do die, medical care is organized either to allow patients "too far gone" to die as comfortably as possible, or to give adequate medical and nursing care to those patients who do not recover despite attempts to save them.

This means that hospitals are already organized "in their fashion" for giving terminal care. Specific hospitals or specific services may not offer very satisfactory care to their dying patients, but provisions for terminal care certainly are built into their organized work. Where adequate or superior terminal care is given, the wards are well supplied with sufficient numbers of skilled personnel, excellent equipment and necessary drugs, plus a division of labor that adequately utilizes those varied resources. Of course, unless the hospital is of a special type that houses mostly patients who will die there, the staff's main concerns will be with "saving" and "recovering," with sending patients home alive and, if possible, in better condition than when they entered the hospital. Nevertheless, as our pages have shown, the personnel may reap many rewards while caring for patients who do die.

Despite the personal satisfactions and the providing of adequate medical resources, few people would claim that terminal care is as good as it could be, and many would argue that it is very deficient on the social-psychological level. Our own position is that the current system is perhaps as good as it can be, but that the system itself needs radical reform. While the best modes of terminal care can be kept, they need to be supplemented by new modes, while both new and old require a different overall organization. The recommendations that we shall offer derive from the unquestionably deficient social and psychological aspects of contemporary terminal care. Taken together with medical and nursing care, they are designed to suggest a new organization of terminal care.

Our recommendations have two main characteristics. First, they are guided by our theory of dying trajectories.[1] Second, they are not offered piecemeal, but as a related series or "package." We believe that tampering with the present system of terminal care

1. The recommendations offered here are based on the research described not only in the present volume but in two other volumes issued by our research team, namely *Awareness of Dying, op. cit.*, and *The Nurse and the Dying Patient* (New York: Macmillan, 1967), by Jeanne Quint.

merely to institute a specific change here and there, without consideration of systematic corrections to the whole system, will do little to improve today's terminal care. Indeed, partial reforms are likely to bring unsuspected consequences that may actually work against improved care. There is need for a systematic, comprehensive, concentrated, and determined effort to reform contemporary modes of caring for the dying.

As an implied critique of current practices, recommendations should be systematic and general, though pointed. They should suggest workable alternatives and capitalize on whatever strengths exist in the present organization. The systematic nature of our inquiry and the integrated character of our theory allow us to sketch, at least, the outlines of reforms that are needed if the care of dying patients and their families is—by almost anyone's standards—to become more compassionate and effective. The recommendations offered here are suggested as first guiding steps, not as a final or definitive formulation of desirable reforms.

RECOMMENDATIONS

1. *Training for giving terminal care should be greatly amplified and deepened in schools of medicine and nursing.*

The training that physicians and nurses receive as students equips them principally for restricted technical aspects of dealing with dying and death. Medical students, for instance, learn not to kill patients through error, and to save patients' lives through diagnosis and treatment; but their teachers put little or no emphasis on how to talk with dying patients, how (or whether) to disclose an impending death, or even how to approach the subject with wives, children and parents of dying patients. Nothing is taught explicitly about the web of social relationships that grows up around a patient who lingers while dying, nor about the reactions of staff when a valued patient dies unexpectedly. Similarly, nursing students are taught how to give nursing care to terminal patients, as well as how to give post-mortem care, but only recently have the "psychological aspects" of nursing care been included in their training. Few teachers talk about such matters, and they generally confine themselves to a lecture or two on "dying," given near the end of the course, sometimes calling in a psychiatrist to give a kind of expert testimony.

Although both doctors and nurses in training do have some experience with dying patients, the emphasis is on the necessary techniques of medicine or nursing, not on the fact of dying itself. This emphasis reflects quite accurately the assumption by the respective faculties that terminal care is primarily a technical matter; its psychological, social and organizational aspects are either secondary or absent. In consequence, most of the behavior of physicians and nurses toward the dying is similar to that of the laymen. Only their more technical behaviors are professionalized.

The clear implication is that medical and nursing curricula should be changed to include the more psychological, social and organizational aspects of terminal care. This is not the place to elaborate those changes in detail, but our critique suggests that the changes need to be fairly extensive. Considerable experimentation will be necessary before faculties can be satisfied that they have provided adequate training in aspects of terminal care now relatively neglected.

Some experimentation will pertain to how and when to teach these matters; the most extensive initial educational turmoil is likely to come from faculty members' own attitudes toward dying and death. These include not only their personal anxieties and aversions to talking openly about dying in any except contemporary technical terms, but also their deep-seated professional attitudes that social, psychological and organizational matters are irrelevant or minor in the cure of illness and the care of patients. In short: the educational reform that we advocate goes beyond merely humanizing the curriculum a little more in order to make terminal care a bit more human.

2. *Explicit planning and review should be given to the psychological, social and organizational aspects of terminal care.*

Our research has demonstrated how strikingly different are the dying trajectories characteristic of different types of wards. There-fore, how very different must be the organizational efforts on each ward to cope with its particular patterns of dying. Although responsible personnel are well aware both of the patterns we have called trajectories, and of organization, they take very little cogni-zance in their planning and review of related matters that are not strictly "nursing" or "medical." The exception occurs only when particular patients or their kinsmen force psychological, social or organizational issues on the staff's attention.

The corrective reform called for is, again, rather radical. Hos-pitals need to make their personnel accountable for many social and psychological actions that currently are left to personal dis-cretion and only incidentally are reported upward—or downward or sideways.

Technical aspects of work are planned, carried out explicitly, reported in writing or orally, and reviewed either by responsible superiors or by colleagues. In contrast, as we have discussed more fully elsewhere,[2] most other actions of personnel toward and around dying patients are nonaccountable. Personnel do and say many things that only incidentally or accidentally reach the eyes and ears of other personnel. The psychological and the social as-pects of terminal care may be good, but they are carried out on the basis of private initiative and judgment rather than as part of accountable decision-making. Although blocking these private actions would be a grave mistake, it does make sense to extend to them the boundaries of accountability.

This means that medical and nursing personnel need to under-stand the characteristic trajectories of dying that occur on their specific wards, not only as medical, but also as organizational and social phenomena. When they have recognized and understood these patterns, there should be explicit planning for coping with them, and provision for reviewing the results. Unquestionably, spe-cial training will be required, for otherwise staff members will not

2. Anselm Strauss, Barney Glaser, and Jeanne Quint, "The Non-Accountability of Terminal Care," *Hospitals,* 38 (January 16, 1964), pp. 73–87.

understand what happens—socially, psychologically, organization-ally—to themselves, or to patients and their relatives during the various stages of characteristic dying trajectories.

No doubt institutional supports will be added. When medical and nursing personnel begin to confront explicitly many problems which they now handle explicitly or ineffectively, they will need considerably more psychological and moral bolstering than is now supplied by the occasional use of psychiatrists and chaplains. Moreover, these men cannot supply the organizational "backstop-ping" which will be required. New organizational mechanisms must be invented. In short, what may be required is the entire reorganization of some services, especially if they deal with high proportions of dying patients.

Quite as urgent is the need for a rational scrutiny of char-acteristic dying trajectories that occur both on new types of wards and when new technologies are introduced to old wards. Each of those innovations brings about new social and organizational "problems" relevant to terminal care. Ordinarily the staff is sensi-tively alert only to their medical or technical features. The giving of adequate nursing and medical care, however, involves a wider orbit of concern and unquestionably requires somewhat different types of ward organization than usually are invented. For instance, kidney transplantation brings about a series of problems involving the patient and the donor and the staff that in turn probably re-quire a somewhat different ward organization than ordinarily has been instituted. This may necessitate new roles for personnel and perhaps even new types of personnel.

In addition, all wards need to develop mechanisms for insur-ing a wider awareness of degrees of agreement and disagreement about what is to be done to, for, and around dying patients. Rarely do personnel agree entirely about these matters and some-times they disagree strikingly, yet they do not always know that they agree or disagree. As our book shows vividly, consensus and dissent are patterned; they are not at all accidental nor independ-ent of phases of a dying trajectory. Each ward needs mechanisms for discovering its patterned disagreements, and for mitigating their destructive impact on the care of patients. It is worth special emphasis that each ward also needs to understand its patterned agreements, for these can also be destructive to medical and nursing care.

3. *There should be explicit planning for phases of the dying trajectory that occur before and after residence at the hospital.*

Most planning for phases outside the hospital is strictly medical, or deals with financial aspects of the patient's life or with matters of geographic mobility. As our chapters have illustrated repeatedly, the illness careers of dying patients take them in and out of hospitals, and adequate terminal care often cannot be given unless the connections between hospital and outside world are explicitly rationalized. Especially is this true for certain types of trajectories in which re-entry is predictable and sometimes repeated. Planning must also take into account the patient's visits to the clinic, for even when he is well enough to stay outside the hospital (as in children's diseases that lead eventually and surely to their death) or infrequently enters the hospital for medical treatment, his clinic visits represent phases of his dying trajectory which currently are regarded either as purely medical matters or as psychologically unconnected with death.

Similarly, the post-mortem phase thrusts the family quickly out of the hospital, where it is left to cope with its grief and its problems either with only its own resources or with the temporary slight aid of funeral personnel. If lucky, surviving relatives may be helped by friends, neighbors, clergymen and compassionate attending physicians. In any event, the hospital's medical and nursing personnel are finished with the family after it leaves the hospital. While many a family would not wish this situation to be changed —once out of the hospital they do not wish to be "reminded," wish no further connection with it—it is also true that many others would welcome professional counsel and perhaps even professional therapy. If the hospital, or some extension of its services, is to minister to family members, then new institutional mechanisms must be developed far beyond the social worker's occasional call, or the infrequent voluntary visit to the hospital by the grateful

relatives. If the hospital takes up these functions, it is also req-
uisite that the families of patients who die at home receive some
professional help during the post-mortem period.

4. *Finally, medical and nursing personnel should encourage*
public discussion of issues that transcend professional responsibili-
ties for terminal care.

This recommendation refers to certain events that repeatedly
occur during dying trajectories and are debated by hospital personnel. These events represent grave problems that are genuinely
unresolvable by the professional community, because they belong
in the public domain. Only when they are debated within the
wider public arena, so that sentiment then develops for certain
solutions, can hospital personnel begin to act in genuinely rational
ways about these issues.

Two problems that we believe need public debate are the
withholding of addicting drugs until "near the end," and the
"senseless prolonging" (personnel's terminology) of life. The first
issue perhaps is the simpler of the two. American attitudes toward
addiction being what they are, there is considerable tendency to
hold back on the addicting drugs even when it can hardly matter
whether a patient who is unquestionably dying will become an
addict. Although there is some disagreement among staff people
about this matter, and certainly some disagreement about the
pacing of such drugs, hospital personnel in general seem to share
the wider public's view of addiction. But this horror of addiction
is not accepted by all Americans, nor would they all be inclined
to sanction the withholding of addicting drugs from dying patients
if this practice were more widely known.

More important, perhaps, is the second issue of "prolonging,"
since modern technology makes increasingly probable the prolonging of lives beyond where patients are capable of appreciating the
extra moments, days or months. Our book, and the others de-
riving from the same research project, have illustrated vividly
how families, as well as staff members, may suffer from the prolonging of life. Debates are frequent within the hospital about
particular evidencies of prolonging. Yet each physician, and occa-

sionally each nurse, must make decisions about particular patients' lives, basing the decision on a sense of professional responsibility combined perhaps with standards of public conscience and sensibility. While the physician and nurse can decide for particular patients, they cannot decide the wider issue. That must be debated by the more general public. With some certainty, one can predict that this issue will increasingly be discussed openly as medical technology becomes increasingly efficient.

CONCLUDING REMARKS

We have made four major recommendations, together with a number of subsumed minor ones. There is, of course, no end to the more specific suggestions that could be made in connection with implementing the major recommendations; indeed we urge readers to think of additional ones with respect especially to their specific institutions.

Our recommendations pertain respectively to the training of professionals, to the reorganization of hospitals, to the relationship of hospitals with the world outside, and to issues that ought to be debated by the lay public. Each recommendation builds on, rather than ignores or simply substitutes for, contemporary modes of providing terminal care. Each major recommendation is linked logically with the other three. There is good reason to think of them as a *set* of recommendations rather than just a random listing. If the present system of providing terminal care is to be much improved, at least in the directions indicated by our research, then it must be improved simultaneously along all the lines of our major recommendations. As we remarked earlier, tinkering with the system, following out one recommendation or another, will not bring about the rational, compassionate care that patients and their families deserve—and from which staff members would also benefit. In sum, a comprehensive reform is required.

Appendix on Method

Our investigation utilized field methods, a complex body of research strategies and techniques that involves direct contact with organizations, groups, and persons under "natural" conditions. Field methods have been used for many years by anthropologists and sociologists, with increasing attention given to the methological problems that are involved in gathering and analyzing data. During the life of our research project, we also have added to the methodological literature. Interested readers can find in *The Discovery of Grounded Theory* (Chicago: Aldine Publishing Company, 1967) detailed discussions of the comparative method and the theoretical sampling on which the present volume is based.

Since this specific methodology is available there for examination, and since our field work did not depart markedly from that discussed in the general literature, this appendix will be short. Its chief purpose is to describe briefly the structural conditions under which the field work was carried out and how those conditions influenced the particular tactics which were either chosen or developed in the field situation. We have chosen this focus chiefly because there is no tradition for systematically linking tactics and structural conditions. Most reports of field work tend to emphasize either the tactics or the setting within which the research occurred, loosely suggesting their connections. We believe a more explicit detailing of the connections might help readers to judge the value of "the evidence."

WORKING CONDITIONS

Suppose one looks first at a few of the central properties of the field in which our research was carried out. The field work was done on the wards of various hospitals, where personnel are somewhat or greatly concerned with the frequently difficult problems of caring for dying patients. For the staff, terminal care is *work,* and this is done in the context of other work. The personnel talk easily and frequently about the dying, and about certain types of daily episodes pertaining to dying and death. They talk about these matters in the context, again, of other talk and in relation mainly to their own work. Moreover, since dying takes time, their conversations and work with the dying vary through time. And since more than one patient may be dying, various combinations of talk and action may occur on successive days and weeks, just as different combinations occur on different types of wards.

These properties make easy and "natural" the use of several field tactics—so much so that the researchers were surprised when laymen, hearing of the study, commented sympathetically about how "difficult" the research must be. By difficult, the commentators sometimes meant difficult "to take" emotionally, but also difficult to "get at." What they did not realize was how much hospital personnel are concerned with problems attending the care of the dying.

A basic field tactic was to show concern for the staff's concern, to show interest not only in the problems of patients but in those of the staff itself. This made "trailing" the personnel a natural maneuver, and direct questioning of them during or after events a perfectly reasonable action. Occasional extensive and frank interviewing had to be linked with our concern for their concern, and the interviews carefully fitted into their work routines. In this kind of setting, there is no great problem in being an available listener and conversationalist, in getting people to talk, being allowed to listen to conversation among colleagues, or watching work done around the patients. Getting and maintaining "rapport," which in other settings sometimes represent major problems, are here relatively easy. Even the problem of gaining entry to the locale is minimized. Nowhere were we refused quick access to it or to most events that we wished to observe.

Among the other central properties of this setting are that the personnel themselves, the private physicians and the more elusive staff physicians, are readily observable on a daily basis. Also the successive events which attend a lengthy dying trajectory enable the researcher to gather data chronologically. He can see events develop over time, and in relation to preceeding events. Also the daily three-shift feature of hospitals makes it easy to note consequences of that feature and also to gain other excellent data, since the work shifts must report to each other verbally and in writing. Similarly, the occasional "days off" taken by various staff members make simpler the observer's task of seeing what difference the presence or absence of various persons may make to the ward's interaction. One more property is especially worth noting: the close proximity of different types of wards, as well as of different types of dying, makes contrasts stand out quickly and vividly, thereby facilitating comparative analysis. In short, many tasks that field workers in other settings find difficult are here rendered easy. No very special tactics are called for in order to gather the desired data.

The problems of "overidentification" or "overinvolvement" with the people being studied were also minimized. Had we closely interviewed patients, these problems might have been severe. Since patients were, for the most part, only observed, the research team discovered to its surprise that the problems of disengagement from the dying were relatively slight. What also helped was that two or three wards were sometimes studied simultaneously, and that prolonged absence from a ward was often possible: both types of discontinuity furthered disengagement, and hence noninvolvement.

TEMPORAL CONDITIONS

On the other hand, the very properties of the setting that provided opportunities raised certain temporal problems for the field workers. Personnel were often extremely busy. While this furthered our observation, it delayed our talking with them about specific events, about which we needed clarification or about which we suspected they had opinions, until another hour or another day. One tactic was to wait for a moment's break, and then "shoot the question." But the opportunity to do so might be long in coming.

Another feature of the wards was also a time-waster: on several days in succession a researcher might discover a given ward had no dying patients. Since he preferred to interview personnel about current patients, the alternative to observe them work with recovering patients was to visit another ward. The fact that each hospital has many kinds of wards considerably minimized wasted time. For this reason he had only to develop relationships with personnel on two or three wards, and then go to a certain ward when on the others nothing much on which we were focused was transpiring or staff was too busy.

On the other hand, this tactic of going to another ward also led, at times, to difficulties. Too many interesting and theoretically relevant events might be occuring simultaneously on two or three wards. This necessitated the priority decision (which frequently confronts the field worker) on where to observe next. He could decide in favor of one ward, but more usually floated between two or three wards, observing selectively according to the emerging theory. (The field workers usually observed in different hospitals, and so could rarely assist one another quickly enough in these observational dilemmas.) "Floating" had to be used even on single wards, for some were quite large. Decisions had to be made whether to follow one trajectory or another, or whether to alternate between them.

Again, the very duration of some trajectories meant that an important event might occur while the observer was absent. This presented no particular hazard unless he was closely following a given trajectory. Then keeping abreast of the news was very important. The appropriate tactic was, when next on the ward, to query personnel about "the latest" in the life of the dying patient.

The length of some trajectories presented other problems involving "timing." Given, say, a trajectory of two weeks, how many days could a researcher afford to be absent from the ward? Some trajectories, after all, spanned weekends. What about the night hours? This kind of problem never was solved satisfactorily. During expected "last hours," the observer attempted to be present if he was vitally interested in the particular trajectory. But the staff's expectation of final hours might be completely wrong, and so research time might be wasted; or, try as he might, the researcher might be unable to be present during those hours. The most general tactic that evolved for handling this difficult matter of timing was to insure a good sampling of the day, evening and night. To that tactic was added another: sampling was guided by our theoretical considerations. Thus, when we needed to know about death watches, we made certain that we were present during *some* of them. In fact, such tactics were immensely supplemented during any given week—to our great relief—by a number of events which were relevant to our concerns. Only this fortunate property of the setting allowed us to solve, to some extent, the problem of being present for the given trajectory at the right place and at exactly the right time.

Lengthy trajectories also subjected the researcher to the same hazards as the staff: weariness and drained emotions. Despite our earlier remarks about minimal identification with patients, a long and difficult dying affected the researcher as well as the personnel. Even without marked identification, the sheer task of following the trajectory—since this involved repeated visits and a great deal of observation and interviewing—could be tiring. The researcher's identification problem was partly solved by his talking to others on the research team, and by his deliberate occasional absences from the ward or simultaneous observations, for relief, on other wards. The weariness that resulted from observing for several days without much break was relieved only to the extent that the researcher rarely needed to be present all day, and could take a holiday from his work after a trajectory had ended.

This brief account of tactics rendered relatively easy or difficult by the structural conditions under which our inquiry was conducted could be greatly expanded. But it must be qualified by two provisos. First, the structured conditions are related to tactics only insofar as both relate to the *inquiry*. Had our research raised different sets of major questions, then different tactics might have been called for—and different or additional structural conditions might have had to be taken into account. Second, when the researcher knows the setting quite well beforehand, then its relevant structural conditions are more or less known in advance. Consequently, appropriate tactics can be worked out in advance. When little is known about the setting, however, the *discovery* of structural conditions and the *inventing* of effective tactics (or "falling into" them) go hand in hand. Even when the institutional terrain is relatively well known—as in our study—there is a reciprocal process of discovering relevant conditions and creating relevant tactics. As our theory about care of the dying evolved, our tactics changed accordingly. Some that were used early in the research were later abandoned, while others became more useful. This continual intermeshing of the conditions of the research and the development of the theory necessitates a constant evolution of tactics —and these tactics, in turn, serve further to develop and elaborate the theory.

Index

CPSIA information can be obtained at www.ICGtesting.com
Printed in the USA
BVOW041256190613

323754BV00001B/114/P